Praise for
BEAUTY'S DIRTY SECRET

"I am a big advocate of natural product use on my site, <u>Liveto110.</u> <u>com</u>. I lecture about the dangers of obesogens, chemicals in personal care products that make us fat and disrupt our hormones. Even many so-called natural products have synthetic, harmful chemicals sneaked into them on the ingredients label. Protecting my health by not putting harmful chemicals on and in my body is really important to me. This is why I use Trina Felber's entire line of Primal Life Organics products—because I KNOW exactly what is in them: all natural, healthy, and organic ingredients. Plus, they work really well, unlike a lot of natural products. I consistently recommend Primal Life Organics products to all my clients and my <u>Liveto110.</u> <u>com</u> readers for this reason. I LOVE Primal Life Organics!"

~Wendy Meyers, Health and Nutrition Coach

"Trina cares! She is sharing her knowledge with you to help you get better results, without the toxins. It's really as simple as that. If you're looking for a natural alternative to skin care, look no further than Trina, she's the best!"

~Nick Nanton, 3-Time Emmy Award Winning Director/Producer and Best-Selling Author

"I have long paid attention to the foods that I eat and the products I use on my body. But this book really opened my eyes to the importance of reading labels on even "natural" skin care products."

~Nicki Violetti, co-owner NorCal Strength and Conditioning

"I am so grateful that I met Trina and read this book. It is not an overstatement to say it may have saved my life or the lives of my loved ones. I had always heard about certain products have chemicals in them that could be harmful, but I never really paid much attention until now. Trina really gives the reader an eye-opening understanding of what *really* is occurring when you come in contact with such chemicals. This isn't just a 'might be happening'; it *is* what is actually occurring, and there is no doubt that little by little it is killing us.

"Since reading this book, I have taken responsibility for myself and for others around me by switching to all organic products. In addition to loving this book, I also enjoy using Primal Life Organics. The products work, and they feel great on my skin. My skin looks younger and I am better physically since I have made the switch. It is also a relief to know that my children will grow up organic, and I have Trina to thank for that!"

~Elena Cardone, Actress,
The G&E Show, Women In Power

"Even if you're super nutrition savvy, you might not know what you put on your skin can become just as harmful or helpful as what you eat. Trina Felber's new book provides smart, effective, Paleo-based strategies for glowing skin, addressing skin conditions, and even a chapter about healthy skin for guys. A must-read."

~JJ Virgin, Celebrity, Nutrition and Fitness Expert

"I am a gluten intolerant mother of a celiac child and I am an actress. Both myself and my children are chemically sensitive beings with allergies to other food such as soy, dairy and artificial food coloring. After switching to a Paleo diet, I couldn't help but notice how much my health and well-being significantly improved. But trying to find a makeup or skin care product on the market that doesn't contain any of these things was almost impossible… Until I found Trina Felber and Primal Life Organics. In this book, Trina will eloquently and passionately educate you to the hidden toxins that comprise your 'natural' shampoos, body lotions, makeup, sunscreens, toothpaste, deodorant. This book taught me that healthy eating is only half the story. If you want true health, you must protect your body's greatest protector…its skin!"

~Leigh-Allyn Baker, Actress, Director,
Executive Producer, *Will & Grace,*
Good Luck Charlie, and *Bad Hair Day*

IT'S TIME TO STOP THE SKIN WAR

If you use big cosmo beauty products, every cell of your body is silently screaming right now. The toxins in our skincare products are quietly wreaking havoc on our bodies and nobody is talking about it. Manufacturers aren't required to label the potions we spend so much money on.

The skin is the body's largest and most vulnerable organ. The absorption of toxins and chemicals through the dermal layer damages our skin cells and creates disease states in the body. You may feed your body healthy, organic, gluten-free food, while toxins are seeping through your skin—destroying your efforts and damaging your internal organs.

This book was written by Trina Felber, RN, BSN, MSN, CRNA. She's a Paleo guru who's dedicated her life to preventing disease through education and real food. Trina is also the owner and creator of Primal Life Organics; a real-food skincare range that feeds the skin the nutrients it needs to function normally.

Beauty's Dirty Secret will show you how to build the beautiful skin you desire using only three simple steps:

- **Ditch the chemical-laden products that are hurting you.**
- **Detox the body by adjusting your skin diet.**
- **Feed your skin the nutrients it needs to thrive and heal yourself from accumulated toxins.**

If healthy eating makes you feel good, then you'll be shocked at the positive effects of the real-food skin diet.

**Featured On:
CBS, ABC, NBC, Fox**

BEAUTY'S DIRTY SECRET

3 Simple Steps to Super Power Your Skin

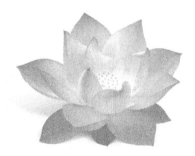

Trina Felber

CEO Primal Life Organics™ , RN, BSN, MSN, CRNA

PLO Publishing LLC

For more information contact:
PLO Publishing LLC
www.primallifeorganics.com

ISBN: 978-0-692-33307-5 Paperback
ISBN: 978-0-692-33308-2 ebook

Library of Congress Control Number: 2014956939

This book is not intended as a substitute for the medical advice of physicians. The reader should regularly consult a physician in matters relating to his/her health and particularly with respect to any symptoms that may require diagnosis or medical attention.

Book design by Dotti Albertine

This book is dedicated to

The air we breathe...
...that you stay as fresh and unpolluted as possible.

The water we drink...
...that you nourish our cells with pure H2O
free from harmful chemicals and pollutants.

The soil we sow...
...that you fill our food with the nutrients
we need to maintain health

My husband Josh...
...without you, this book would still be in my head
and not on paper. Thank you for your support,
guidance, love and patience. I am grateful we share the
same passion for life, health and thinking outside the box.

My children, Mia, Cash and Roman...
...that you may have fresh air to breathe, clean water
to drink and nutrient rich soil to grow your food.
You give my life meaning and purpose,
and Primal Life Organics™ was created so
you could be given the healthiest start in life.

...My parents, Suzanne and Roger Prucnal
...for inspiring me to be creative, think outside the box
and to never stop believing in myself.

...My sisters, Leslie Schubargo, Valerie Brown,
Adriann Finkler and Libby Sorosiak
...for being sisters and sharing the same passion
for health and beauty that I do. For testing my
creations, honest feedback and lots of laughs!

...Rebecca Stoneman
...my mother-in-law. For your love of nature and
your continued and unwavering support
of all I have created.

I dedicate this book to every cell of every tissue
of every organ of every system of every body.
That you may live in a toxin free environment
and enjoy a toxic free life-span.

———————

Trina Felber
CEO and Creator, Primal Life Organics™
RN, BSN, MSN, CRNA
Wife, Mother, Health Enthusiast,
Paleo Advocate and Cavegirl

Contents

Foreword

*B*ig Cosmo keeps a secret. Those tiny, expensive and exquisite jars of lotions, potions and serums promise to do big things. But what's on the inside is what matters. And what's inside those tiny, beautiful bottles? A dirty secret.

Mother Nature holds within her realms a few dirty little secrets of her own. I discovered Mother Nature's dirty little secret… and I will share it with you. I am going to reveal the truths that have been hidden from you and let you decide how you want to feed your skin.

Stop The Skin War.

I spent hours and hours at the Big Cosmo cosmetic departments. I have spent thousands of dollars on beauty potions promising clear, younger looking, beautiful skin. I am where I am today because Big Cosmo never came through with its promises. I searched for reasons my skin was acne infested, oily, and aging in spite of my expensive skincare. What I discovered was the truth Big Cosmo didn't want me to know.

When I became savvy enough to read the labels, I instantly knew Big Cosmo was POISONING me with cheap chemicals that were causing harm to my entire being. Every cell of my body was silently screaming. **Becoming pregnant made me realize using these chemicals was NOT a risk I was willing to take.** How much is too much? Big Cosmo would have you believe its lab-made chemicals are safe. I beg to differ. A cancer-causing chemical is a cell mutagen. Even a little is too much for me! I realized that the only way to heal the body (both inside and out) is through real food.

I ditched processed foods, wheat, gluten and dairy, and did so in my skincare as well. It wasn't until I discovered real food through my diet and how it healed my body that I began to question the intentions of Big Cosmo. When I started to listen to my body, I realized that my BODY was telling me, "I want real food!" That was the emphatic chant ringing through my body. When I changed my skin-diet to real food, I saw RESULTS! Real food is what the body craves, and the skin is no different.

So, I created my own line of skincare using only real food sources, and what I discovered shocked me. My skin LOVED it! The results I longed for from my high priced lotions never happened, but when I applied food to my face and body, my oiliness, acne and psoriasis disappeared. I was left with skin others crave! I longed for healthy skin for so long, it looked even better in person!

Recently, numerous individuals have told me that I look to be in my late 20s-early 30s! They are blown away when I tell them I am 46 years young!

"Put food on your skin," I tell them, "and you will SEE the results you crave!"

I have become a leading Expert in creating real food options for commercial skincare. I created Primal Life Organics in 2012, and set out to market my company as a leader in the skincare industry that uses only real food sources for ingredients meant to DETOX, FEED, HEAL and PROTECT the body. What I found was hundreds, now thousands of men and women that have been searching for the same healing, nourishing and protecting that I can offer.

Everyone is searching for ways to improve their health. They are opening their eyes to the real dangers of *processed* foods and skincare. When you find me, **you** feel a sense of relief… like you are HOME!

I make approximately 45 different products including facial care (acne, anti-aging, dry and oily skin variations), body care, hair care, dental care, and makeup. Yes, all made from ingredients Mother Nature gives us.

I am a Certified Registered Nurse Anesthetist therefore I completely understand the physiology of the body. Until now, I was in a chemical trance. Duped by Big Cosmo—but no longer! I have taken the POWER back! Now, I put the POWER of healing your body in your hands!! I uncover the Great Skin Lie we have been told and teach you how to **super power your skin back to health with the radiant glow you've always wanted!**

You are just three simple steps away from the skin you have always wanted!

Trina Felber

CHAPTER ONE

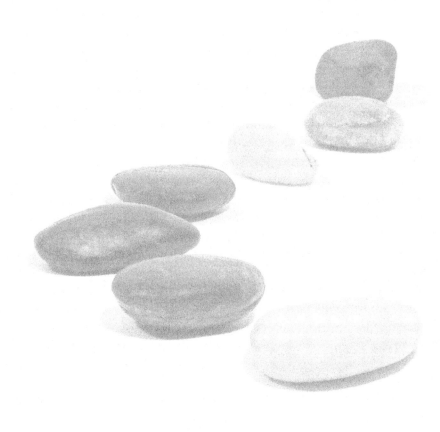

The Great Skin Lie

If you wouldn't eat it, don't put it on your skin. Your skin is your first line of defense, but also the easiest way for toxins to enter your body and pollute your entire system.

What's a protective elastic wrap, strong enough to prevent entry by foreign elements but equally strong at throwing out malignant ones? That is capable of both cooling and warming? And that simultaneously contains and repels water?

Your skin, that's what! Your skin is your body's largest organ. Many of us take great care to eat whole, organically grown, or sustainably raised foods. We do it because we care about what our cells and tissues are made of, and because we know that toxic chemicals are not a part of that picture. We pay more, think harder, and are more selective than the vast majority of consumers.

We pay attention—to the inside.

What many of us never consider is that our amazing skin, the stuff that adorns, defends and houses us, is also a mighty vehicle for absorbing both nutrients and toxins. Most women—and increasingly more men—use daily cosmetics, lotions, cleansers, and enhancers they've carefully selected from their trusted natural products providers. But what we don't know about what composes these "natural" products can seriously harm us.

I spent thousands of dollars purchasing skincare that promised RESULTS such as; younger looking, clear, less wrinkles, and even skin tone. Did I ever see any results? NO. Did I go back for more? YES. Why? I wanted to believe Big Cosmo was selling the same "miracle cream" that they had advertised so well. I trusted Big Cosmo. I believed they would not put ingredients in my skincare that could cause harm to me, or my developing baby. What I discovered was the Great Skin Lie. Big Cosmo was not protecting me. They were more concerned with mass-producing products as cheap as possible. Using unfiltered water, chemical preservatives, and lab made toxins that cause more harm to my body than I ever gave one thought to. The beautiful woman in the white lab coat probably has no idea what phthalates are, or how they disrupt my endocrine system. Truth is, I never gave Big Cosmo the permission to poison me!

It wasn't until I discovered real food through my diet and how it healed my body that I began to question the intentions of Big Cosmo. When I started to listen to my body, I realized what my BODY was telling me "I want real food!" It was the emphatic chant ringing through my body. When I changed my skin-diet to real food, I saw RESULTS! Real food is what the body craves, and the skin is no different.

Early in my skincare journey, I remember reading an article that brought to light a British report that estimated women who use makeup soak in about five pounds of cosmetic chemicals each year. It was my first taste of these studies—they all highlighted what to know about beauty products before diving in and making a purchase. The average American uses about ten different personal care products a day, which can quickly add up to a hundred different chemicals . . . this is problematic, troublesome, and dangerous when you consider that "more than one-third of all personal care products contain at least one ingredient linked to cancer," according to the Environmental Working Group (EWG). Never mind the ingredients linked to birth defects.

This horrendous and scary news is the main reason I develop products made from natural, organic, earthen, Paleo ingredients. I want to enjoy my golden years healthy, not fighting a cancer I could have prevented by avoiding toxic chemicals.

Another Great Skin Lie: Manufacturers are not required to put warning labels on skincare products. The product label may say "natural," and many of the elements used may be naturally derived, but more often than not, they are combined with others we seldom know about. Some of the most innocuous elements often found in natural products are either downright bad or counterproductive to the cosmetic's purpose.

Most natural products are scented, but manufacturers aren't required to list or differentiate the components of the fragrance on the label. Their fragrance blend is proprietary to the company—a trade secret. But many fragrance components also happen to be neurotoxins. They have the ability to cross the placental barrier during pregnancy, causing birth defects and DNA damage. They can also affect learning, concentration, digestion, and reproduction. These changes are minute and happen over time, so it is very difficult for us to connect our skin conditions, bloating, sluggishness, slowed metabolism, and other health issues with our skincare regimen.

What does slowed metabolism mean to most people? Weight gain. Our culture is in the throes of an obesity problem that could very well be connected to toxins in our diets and products. The ingredients in your skincare can influence and impair your thyroid-gland function. A malfunctioning thyroid can slow your metabolism and cause weight gain. Weight gain (especially as we age) typically includes increasing amounts of fat cells. More fat cells (adipose tissue) allow for increased storage of toxins and chemicals from all sources, including the environment, our diet, and skincare products. We will discuss how all of this is possible in Chapter Four.

Who knew that water can be dehydrating? I didn't, until I began my investigative research on the components of not just cosmetics, but "natural" cosmetics and skincare products. What I found was that water—often listed as a primary ingredient in natural products—is used to increase volume and decrease the amount of the actual product that nourishes your skin. Yet, as it dries, water pulls moisture out of the skin. Furthermore, the water added to skincare products is *regular, polluted tap water*. We live in a society that pays top dollar for filtered drinking water, yet we slather our largest organ with polluted tap water.

Trying to combine water with the essential oils in most natural products is futile—water and oil don't mix. It's science. Therefore, in order to make them mix, an emulsifier must be added to the mix and wouldn't you know—most emulsifiers are harmful to the body.

Tapioca starch is often used as an emulsifier in healthy cosmetics. But tapioca starch contains gluten, and gluten is an allergen. Many people never consider that though they may eliminate gluten from their diets, if their cosmetics still contain wheat, barley, oats, or rye, then they are still absorbing gluten, which can in turn cause a multitude of problems. Hair products, too, are often manufactured with gluten-containing components. Absorbing gluten through the skin can be key to celiacs who maintain a gluten-free diet, but still struggle with irritable bowel syndrome (IBS).

While I was pregnant with my first child and living a very healthy lifestyle, I discovered that not only were my "natural" products not actually 100 percent natural, but also they could potentially affect my growing fetus in a very negative way (more on that later). As a Certified Registered Nurse Anesthetist, I used my science background to begin developing skincare products that I could safely use during my pregnancy and beyond. From my Paleo diet perspective, I chose the healthiest components possible and discovered that applying whole foods to your skin means getting many of their benefits, including vitamins and minerals, through absorption. One by one, I developed the skincare products that now comprise my Primal Life Organics line.

My family and I are living, breathing examples of the benefits of the Paleo (often called Primal) diet, and our experience with organic living has convinced me that there is no healthier way to live. My products are based on my firm belief that whole foods have the ability to nourish not only the inside of your body, but the outside as well. If you're reading this book, you may already be eating Paleo. Or maybe you don't yet, but have heard how good of a lifestyle change it might be for you. Even if you're not Paleo diet adherent, you probably picked up this book because you want to know more about how to make changes in your lifestyle that can feed, nourish, and protect your healthy body and spirit.

The Paleo diet means eating only those foods that our ancestors, the cavemen, ate. Some health-focused people are uncomfortable with the idea of a Primal diet because they don't understand that it just means consuming only whole foods (meats, vegetables, nuts, berries, and fruits), while eliminating gluten and dairy. Many people reading this book already have great diets and are only one small dietary change away from eating strictly Paleo.

I took the Paleo diet a step further by melding real foods with natural elements into a line of skincare products that are freshly made to order, with zero preservatives, emulsifiers, or artificial fragrances. Paleo is synonymous with real food. I put only real food on my skin. Nothing contaminated with chemicals or toxins. Nothing processed, artificial or lab-made. My skin glows because the cells are nourished and can eliminate toxins instead of accumulate them. I decongested my skin, and I will share with you the benefits of providing real food for your skin so you can reap the benefits that I have seen. Look at what you currently use and see if those products contain any of the toxic items I mention in Chapter Four. Then look at Chapter Five and you'll see why the fresh, quality ingredients I choose to use are so incredibly important.

I am an *advocate for prevention* and I'm sure this stems from my twenty-year nursing career, advocating for patients who are either too sick to advocate for themselves, or not educated enough to know better. I extend that commitment to my skincare business. I converted my passion into my business. I made my skincare for myself, I created my company so you could have healthy skincare options too. Primal Life Organics is my way of advocating for you and your family.

There are numerous, uncontrollable cancer-causing variables in our everyday life. Some are truly unavoidable. But more importantly, some are VERY PREVENTABLE.

I understand that organic, natural skin care can be more costly, but inviting cancer that could have been prevented is far more costly in so many ways (physically, emotionally, and financially) for both you and your loved ones. Please don't misread this—I am not saying if you use organic, natural, Paleo products you will live a cancer-free life. However, I can say that your chances of living a cancer-free life are greater if you avoid slathering your skin with cancer-causing chemicals. You may not lose five pounds on the scale, but this five-pound chemical loss just might improve the quality of your life without you even knowing it—and that is the best loss to win!

This book is about common skin complaints and how whole, real food skincare products can heal them. It's about rubbing the purest lotion onto your growing baby belly and giving your child more nutrients at the same time. It's about assuring that you have what I didn't have when I was first pregnant with my daughter—a line of products that not only make you look and feel good but that do so without compromising your or your baby's health and development.

Welcome to eye-opening knowledge that give you the power to choose. Don't let Big Cosmo keep you in a chemical trance. Wake up—detoxify your skin and body. A chemical free life is awaiting you and NOW you have the POWER to take CONTROL back! Don't let Big Cosmo pollute your body anymore. Wake up to the Great Skin Lie you have been told.

I received my Infiniti Primal Face Package last week. I just want to tell you that I just threw away ALL of the various chemical-laden skincare products I own. I will never use anything else. I am absolutely amazed how good my skin looks after using your products for less than a week. I am stunned. It is like my skin just devours the oils and nutrition in your products. I am not kidding when I say my skin has never looked so good.

—Peggie L.

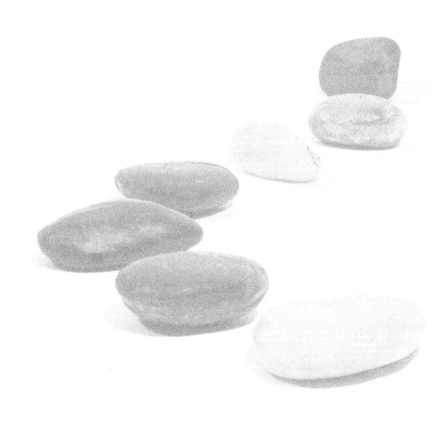

CHAPTER TWO

We Never Gave Big Cosmo Permission to Poison Us

I read the ingredient label of the high-priced moisturizer I was applying to my face, and my hand froze in horror. What are all these things?

I was seven weeks pregnant—the same point at which my last baby had miscarried, sadly, only ten weeks earlier. Of course I was a little nervous and constantly wondered if the miscarriage had been my fault, if it could have been prevented, and what, if anything, I should do now so this baby would make it to be healthy and whole.

I can remember looking in the bathroom mirror and applying my expensive moisturizer. I clearly can see my hand touching my face and freezing, as I just so happened to glance at the ingredients for the first time:

Key Ingredients:

Aloe barbadensis, Pomegranate sterols, Urea, Pistachio nut oil (Pistacia vera), Sodium PCA, Vitamin E (tocopheryl acetate)

Other Ingredients:

Water (Aqua), C12-15 Alkyl Benzoate, Caprylic/Capric Triglyceride, Glyceryl Stearate, Cetearyl Alcohol, Butyrospermum Parkii (Shea Butter), Butylene Glycol, Aloe Barbadensis Leaf Juice, Urea, Sodium Behenoyl Lactylate, Glycerin, Pistacia Vera (Pistachio) Seed Oil, Helianthus Annuus (Sunflower) Seed Oil, Methyl Gluceth-10, Punica Granatum Sterols, Sodium PCA, Glycine, Alanine, Proline, Serine, Threonine, Lysine, Arginine, Glutamic Acid, Sorbitol, Betaine, Dimethicone, Tocopheryl Acetate, Tocopherol, Disodium EDTA, Fragrance (Parfum), Chlorphenesin, Methylparaben, Propylparaben

My trained nurse's eye instantly identified a few harmful ingredients but most of the others I didn't recognize. *What are those?* I remember thinking. As a self-proclaimed science lover with a masters in nursing, I have to say I found it odd that even I couldn't understand—much less pronounce—the majority of the ingredients that I was thoughtlessly applying to my skin day in and day out.

I was horrified! I not only knew that the skin is the largest organ of the human body, but I had a full understanding that the nutrients and chemicals absorbed through the skin go directly into the bloodstream, cells, and other, less obvious organs. I also knew, from my graduate study of anesthetics, that most chemicals are lipophilic (*fat* loving), meaning that they migrate to and are stored in fatty tissue. One of our most fatty organs also houses our personality,

intelligence, decisions, memory, and mental state—**the brain!**
What could possibly happen if we "overdose" on chemicals and toxins that get stored in our brain? Or in our baby's brain?

Suddenly, it dawned on me: That top-of-the-line, natural product that I had been using for years without ever stopping to question
what was in it, had actually left me with years of accumulated toxins
built up in my body. And now, I was horrified to realize, these same
chemicals were becoming part of my developing baby's body, too.

I grabbed my expensive "all natural" face wash (specially
designed for oily skin) and found Glycerin, Ascorbic Acid, Sesa-
mum Indicum (Sesame) Seed Oil, C12-15 Alkyl Benzoate, Sodium
Cocoyl Isethionate, Hydrogenated Soybean Oil, Sodium C14-16
Olefin Sulfonate, Vitis Vinifera (Grape) Seed Extract, Ginkgo Biloba
Leaf Extract, Panax Ginseng Root Extract, Stearyl Glycyrrhetinate,
Phospholipids, Butylene Glycol, Carbomer, Silica, Fragrance (Par-
fum), Titanium Dioxide (CI 77891).

No way was I going to put that on my skin! I washed my face
with plain (some might consider boring) water and checked my
husband's moisturizer, only to discover another chemical brew.
Down I went to the kitchen for simple olive oil—the only moisturizer I could think of that wouldn't be a toxic soup just waiting to
harm my growing baby.

I looked suspiciously at my top-of-the-line foundation, blush,
eyeliner, and mascara. Every "natural" cosmetic product in my bathroom seemed to rear its ugly chemical head at me. In the end I was
too afraid to look at the ingredients, and just went to work that day
without applying any makeup.

What was Big Cosmo up to? Why so many chemicals? Why polluted water? Am I in a chemical trance, a topically drug-induced

state that only leaves me wanting more? I was not seeing results, yet I kept going back for the same chemical brew. Is my sluggishness, slowed metabolism, frequent ailments, eczema, excessively oily skin, even my miscarriage, somehow related to this chemical intrusion? What could I possibly be like if I detoxed?

In my quest to find truly natural products, I began researching the chemicals in cosmetics and skin care. My first reaction was horror, but my second could only be described as anger at being deceived. How could they put these harmful ingredients into "natural" products without disclosing possible side effects? And what about Big Cosmo? The chemical soup in the cosmetic industry's commercial skincare is one of the most potent. I never gave Big Cosmo permission to poison me!

My thoughts circled around my own unborn baby and the millions of other babies in the bellies of well-intentioned mothers who believed they were using the healthiest, most natural products. I considered my mysterious miscarriage. I thought of the vulnerability of developing fetuses. Could there be a correlation between the multitude of escalating health issues and the number of chemicals we're exposed to every day? Could there be a correlation between these chemicals and the rising levels of obesity in adults *and children?* After all, children—especially infants—may be more susceptible to the harmful toxic effects because of their larger body surface of fat that more readily absorbs everything, and their immature metabolic and elimination systems may be affected or slowed.

I began to ask, "Why are there no warnings on skincare?" Why don't products we put on our skin require the same warnings as foods we put into our bodies? Why do we not see any of these warnings?

Caution: Do not use when pregnant.

Caution: Do not use if trying to avoid cancer.

Caution: Do not use if diabetic.

Caution: Do not use if trying to lose weight.

Caution: Do not inhale.

Caution: Do not use if you have celiac, diarrhea, IBS, or GI malfunction.

Caution: Contains ingredients that irritate and cause skin conditions.

Caution: Contains ingredients that can cause infertility, reproductive problems, birth defects, learning disabilities, concentration problems, early puberty, or DNA damage.

Caution: Do not use if suffering from acne. This could actually be on every acne treatment product that contains benzoyl peroxide. The MSDS—Material Safety Data Sheets—warns benzoyl peroxide is a possible tumor promoter and may act as a mutagen that produces DNA damage. It is toxic by inhalation as well as being an eye, skin, and respiratory irritant. Skin irritants can cause acne, rosacea, and rashes.

I was shocked and dismayed by what I discovered: the cosmetic industry is not required to test their products for safety before they go on the market. On average, children are exposed to more than 50 chemicals every day in the personal care products developed to keep them clean, smelling sweet, and looking good. I can only imagine how many chemicals are part of little babies' cells and tissues just because their mothers unknowingly used chemical-laden "natural" products.

These discoveries made me get serious about researching what truly natural ingredients I could use to have radiant, glowing, healthy skin. I expanded the old adage, "You are what you eat" to include, "You are what you put on your skin." To me, "natural" means whole, organic, *real* food—vegetables, fruits, nuts and nut butters, vegetable oils, naturally occurring clays, and dyes. I used my background in science to formulate and experiment with assorted recipes for my face and body. And I was finally able to relax in the knowledge that what went on my body was also good for my baby growing within it.

At the time, I had *really* oily skin and acne that covered my forehead and jaw. But nothing big, red, and juicy was on my face—just hundreds of little bumpy breakouts that took up residence years earlier and never said good-bye. Imagine my surprise when my skin cleared up over time and reverted to normal. Today, the scars from years of happily picking zits are so faint only I know they're there. And now I often get comments about my beautiful skin and how it glows.

I knew I couldn't change what I'd eaten or used in the past, but I could change the way my health was going now. Using cosmetics and skincare products composed of 100 percent real foods healed my skin, brightened my hair, gave me more energy, and fed my baby from the outside as well as from the inside.

In the wake of my horror and outrage at the chemical industry's callous zeal to increase its profits by polluting our bodies with untested products, I created a healthful and nourishing line of products I call Primal Life Organics Skin-Food. No chemicals, no disguised carcinogens, no DNA disruptors—just simple, effective, and entirely natural goodness for your and your family's health.

This book will help you understand why real food products matter in your life, how to detox from the chemical invasion of the Big Skin Lie, what to feed your skin, and how healing will happen when nutrients replace chemicals in your cells. You'll be surprised by some of my discoveries that may seem counter intuitive (let's put oil on your oily skin!). And you'll discover that toddlers aren't the only ones who can enjoy putting food on their faces.

Trust me when I say I have tried EVERYTHING and am very familiar with high-end products. I HAVE NEVER HAD RESULTS WITH ANYTHING UNTIL I CAME ACROSS Primal Life Organics! I am amazed at the instant change in my complexion. I know you refer to your products as Paleo Skin-Food, but I am here to tell you I call it PALEO SKIN-CRACK!!! My skin LOVES it and wants more! I have no idea how you do it, but PLEASE never stop making this stuff! My skin has never, ever looked this fresh, clear, bright and toned. PALEO SKIN-FOOD is incredible, like no other and totally worth the money! Thanks, Trina, for the amazing Paleo skincare!

—Sunny

CHAPTER THREE

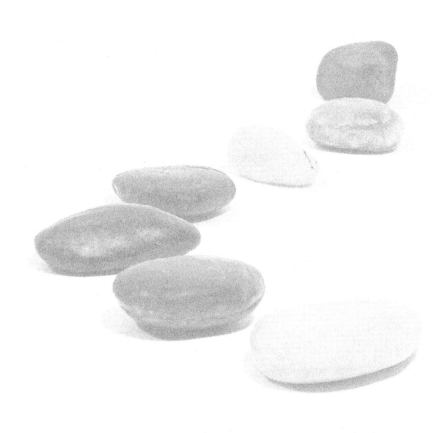

The Nurse's Journey to Discovering the Hidden Truth

I am an experienced nurse who understands the negative effects of neurotoxins and endocrine disruptors very well. But when I realized there were no pure skincare products out there, my research for alternatives began in earnest.

Growing up in Toledo, Ohio, put me in the middle of the country's heartland, while growing up with four sisters put me in the heartland of skincare and beauty products. Because of this, is it any surprise I found a way to help the world through skincare made from wholesome food and dirt (clay)?

I was always health conscious and science driven, even as a young person. In high school I was an intellectual who was curious about the elements, vitamins, minerals, liquids, gases, and solids of science. I was a girl who excelled in math. My desire to help others made the study of human anatomy and physiology particularly fascinating, as I imagined all I could do to relieve pain and suffering in people. During high school I knew medicine would end up becoming my career, and in 1992 I received my RN degree from St. Vincent Medical Center in Toledo.

Having a Type A personality, I immediately wanted to experience the most intense areas of the hospital. For this reason I wound up working as a nurse in the Burn ICU, Medical ICU, and Surgical ICU. These units each dealt with severe, complicated medical issues that challenged my scientific knowledge and nursing expertise. More than that, however, they gave me optimal opportunities to do what I had set out to do: ease pain and suffering. Ten years later I became a traveling nurse and found myself working in the Neuro ICU of Duke University Hospital.

I decided to return home to get my bachelor of science in nursing (BSN), and I attended the University of Akron. Coupling more than a decade of intense nursing experience with advanced scientific training, I received my master of science in nursing (MSN) and became a Certified Registered Nurse Anesthetist in 2007. Though my time spent in hospitals has been affected by the creation of my business, I do still continue to work as a Certified Registered Nurse Anesthetist to this day.

I met my husband and rock, Josh, at a cookout. It quickly became apparent that we shared mutual interests in healthy lifestyles and pure foods, and consequently were instantly drawn to one another. But we also found that we shared similar views on personal fitness, financial goals, and attaining our dreams through hard work and individual responsibility. By the end of 2007, we had flown to Fiji and were married.

We had already been living what we thought was a healthy lifestyle when Josh began to explore the Paleo diet. In 2010, he opened CrossFit Akron and introduced me to the CrossFit training method.

I went into overdrive in an attempt to perfect my personal training, strength, and health, but when it came down to it, his interest in the Paleo lifestyle was what really changed our lives.

Josh didn't need to convince me about its benefits—of which there are many—I immediately saw the rational science in the Paleo diet theory. Before I chose to commit to it completely, however, I used my medical knowledge to extensively research everything about it until the birth of our twin sons, when we decided to live our lives 100 percent Paleo.

Quickly defined, on the Paleo diet, you eat only what our caveman (and cavewoman) ancestors ate—meat and fish, raw or cooked vegetables and fruits, fungi, eggs, roots, and nuts. No dairy or dairy products, processed oils, grains or legumes, potatoes, refined salt or refined sugar. Paleo simply means eating only real foods. I'll talk more about the importance of Paleo in later chapters.

My daughter, Mia, was born in 2008; it was during my pregnancy with her that I had my aha moment regarding the multitude of toxins that are present in "natural" skincare products. Pregnant and searching for "healthy" options, I felt betrayed by Big Cosmo. I felt polluted and poisoned. I felt I had lost control over what went on my body. I felt stripped of my autonomy and power. Because of my training in nursing, I am deeply knowledgeable about the neurotoxins, drugs, nutrients, and chemicals that pass through our skin and enter directly enter our bloodstreams. When I realized I would have to create my own moisturizer if I was going to have one totally free of toxic chemicals, my research into toxins and their effects intensified. I got serious about detoxifying every aspect of my life. Everything, from the food we ate to the cleaning products we used, to the personal hygiene and skincare that went on our skin, it all had to be 100 percent natural.

I created a moisturizer for myself called Carrot Seed. This moisturizer is what made me decide that I wanted to be able to offer this same product purity to other people. In 2008, I began manufacturing natural skincare products under the name Olive's Organic Botanicals.

At that time, we weren't eating totally Paleo. We still ate gluten and dairy, but the more Josh read about it, the closer we came. After our twins, Cash and Roman, were born in 2010, we stopped eating gluten and dairy and wholeheartedly adopted the diet. Right after Josh and I committed to a pure Paleo diet and lifestyle, I realized my skincare products were in line with it.

Even though the Paleo movement was growing quickly, I found no mention of Paleo skincare. As a nurse, it didn't make sense to me to ignore the nutritional value of the products we put on our skin. My thought was, "Surely there are other people eating Paleo who want personal hygiene products that are in line with their dietary standards. What's the point of putting good stuff *in* your body and bad stuff *on* it?" I expanded the Paleo theory of what should be put into your body to include raw, organic, and gluten-free products that went *on* your body, as well.

By 2012, Primal Life Organics Skin-Food was born.

My theory was proven when only six months later Primal Life Organics was a thriving, growing company. Clearly, a need existed for good, quality, fresh, skincare products that are nutrient-dense and moisturizing at the same time.

It's amazing what real food does for the skin. Clarity. Purity. Detoxification. The hunger was there for real food—it was just suppressed by the chemicals that invaded my body and altered the way the cells of my skin could respond. It was dehydrated—but forced to over-produce sebum making me believe it was really oily.

My skin was dazed and confused by the congestion caused by toxic pollutants. Once I changed my skin diet to real food, something magical happened. My skin could talk to me again. It could tell me what it wants—and what it wants is real nutrients. Vitamins, minerals, essential fatty acids, antioxidants are the REAL anti-aging nutritional powerhouses. *Mother Nature knows beauty.* Mother Nature had it right all along. Our ancestors knew what was best for their skin. Big Cosmo changed all of that and made me believe what my skin really needed was "altered."

Not anymore. I took a step back in time. To a time when Mother Nature offered her solutions. I rejected Big Cosmo because nature had it right all along. My skin has never looked better. In fact, feeding the skin real food typically results in very fast and noticeable changes. Dehydrated skin shows wrinkles. Take away the chemicals, (polluted) water and irritants and the skin plumps to life. Hydrated skin will always look younger than dehydrated skin. Anti-aging does not come from a lab. In fact, most lab-made chemicals that Big Cosmo promotes in their anti-aging potions will actually potentiate aging, because of the dehydration and cellular damage they cause.

Many people use products from my Primal Life Organics line, and not all of them do it because they live Paleo. People use these products because they work—they heal, replenish, nourish, and stimulate the skin while giving the entire body a supplemental dose of vitamins and minerals.

My family and I now live a totally Paleo lifestyle—inside and out. From my nurse perspective, it is the absolute best way to raise my children and keep my family's health at its very peak.

And, really, how could I offer anything less than that to the people who trust me with their skin?

Let me give you an inside look at what's happening in your body now and how it will change when you give it pure nutrients instead of toxins. The current picture is downright scary, but your body's future can be a lot better.

Get ready to take the *first step* to Super Power your skin. Ditch the chemicals! Here's why...

_____

I have been using Trina's products for about 8 weeks now and my skin is absolutely glowing!!! My first package was the Infiniti Anti-Aging package (because duh, no one likes wrinkles!). I really love this line of skincare and can't get enough! I have had problems with my skin for years now and have been rescued by this line. It's incredible!

—Amy

CHAPTER FOUR

How Your Skincare Is Making You Fat, Sick, Forgetful and Big Cosmo Money

Toxins and chemicals cause inflammation. Inflammation leads to poorly functioning organs and disease. Disease of any kind stresses the body and ignites the fight or flight response. This vicious cycle leads to slowed metabolism and a host of other health problems. Step one to Super Power Your Skin is to ditch the chemicals. Becoming aware of what is entering your body gives you the power of choice and freedom. Ditching the chemicals allows your body to return to a natural state of being and function. This chapter reveals the secrets Big Cosmo does not want you to know: how they are polluting your body with cheap chemicals that make you fat, sick forgetful and them lots of money.

Modern life on most of planet Earth is *polluted*. Everything—from the water and air to the soil and light—contains ever-increasing concentrations of toxic particles from the manufacture, use, and disposal of the more than 67,317 man-made chemicals from which many of our daily needs are met.

And these are only the disclosed ones. The total number of chemicals affecting our lives is unknown. Most of them have never been tested for their effects on our long-term health or on the environment.

Is it any surprise that rates of asthma, respiratory disease, lung damage, cardiovascular disease, bone weakness, brain disturbances, and cancers of every kind are skyrocketing? Healthcare costs are expected to be one-fifth of the US Gross Domestic Product (GDP) by 2021.[1] Our immune systems are compromised, our cardiovascular systems are overtaxed and weak, our ability to metabolize and regulate is distorted, and more than a third of the US population is obese.[2]

Many of these conditions are the consequences of our biology being assaulted by unnatural and often destructive chemicals. Toxins cause a wide range of changes in our bodies; many chemical effects happen subtly and over time.

Do you associate breathing with weight gain? Consider this: the average human breathes 17,280 times *a day*. Every one of those breaths carries toxic chemicals from the air like ammonia, sulfur dioxide, ozone, lead, and nitrogen dioxide into the lungs and bloodstream. These accumulate in our fat, causing slow but sure damage to multiple body systems, including—and especially—the endocrine system.

Our endocrine system affects every organ and cell in our body and it regulates our metabolism. It controls central development and metabolic processes. When the body doesn't metabolize efficiently, it slows, allowing fat to accumulate more easily.

Chemicals from the body products we use are absorbed through our skin, teeth, gum tissue, scalp, mucous membranes, and

1 http://www.kaiserhealthnews.org/Daily-Reports/2012/June/13/health-care-costs.aspx
2 http://www.cdc.gov/obesity/data/adult.html

respiratory tract. These chemicals that prolong a product's shelf life, emulsify water with oil, promise to make us look younger, heal a skin condition, or stop us from sweating are contributing to the rise in obesity of adults and children by damaging our endocrine systems.

When we eat foods with chemicals, they pass through the liver (a phenomenon called "first-pass") almost immediately after they are digested. The liver metabolizes these chemicals into a water-soluble format. The kidneys excrete the majority of these chemicals through urine (another reason to drink lots of filtered water!). This does not mean it is OK to eat chemically preserved, genetically altered, or hormone-injected food sources just because your liver is your gatekeeper to toxin removal. The liver can be overburdened as well, and an overburdened liver cannot function properly. So keep eating from the perimeter of the grocery store where the good stuff is—fruits, vegetables, grass-fed or local sourced meats, freshwater fish, and unprocessed foods. Your liver will thank you!

Most chemicals are lipophilic, meaning that they are attracted to fat and are easily stored there. Chemicals that are *absorbed by the skin or oral tissue* instead of through the digestive system are deposited directly into the bloodstream and reach all of your organs *before they get to the liver.* This means these fat-loving chemicals do not pass through the liver to be broken down and neutralized before reaching critical organs (like the brain) and tissues. In fact, very few of the chemicals in skincare may ever reach the liver. Most will be absorbed by the organs and fatty tissue and may be stored there for years, inflicting microscopic cellular changes over that time.

You will read more about detoxification in Chapter Five, but for now please understand that the metabolism of skincare chemicals absorbed by the skin is a completely different process than the metabolism of the chemicals ingested from food.

Ingesting chemicals and toxins via skincare is far more dangerous than eating them.

Phthalates, parabens, SLS, benzoyl peroxide, petroleum—to name a few—are all lipophilic. When these endocrine disrupters, DNA mutagens, and carcinogens enter the body through the skin, they are absorbed directly into the bloodstream. They DO NOT go to the liver for dilution and breakdown; they go directly to your vital organs first—full strength! Because they love fatty tissue, they tend to be absorbed by subcutaneous and visceral (organ) fat. Your brain is made up of a large percentage of fat and these chemicals can target your brain.

The small percentage of them that make it to your liver will be broken down and excreted. But the vast majority stays in your adipose (fat) and visceral tissue for years, causing unseen but very REAL damage including reproductive problems, cancer, and decreased thyroid function.

The thyroid hormone is critical to brain, inner ear, and bone development. In adults it is critical to heart function. It also regulates your metabolism. Slow it down through toxic stress, and you could accumulate more fat tissue. Your skincare may be contributing to your weight gain!

Lead is an extremely toxic, very common chemical. Lead contamination comes from any number of sources in the air, food, paint, water, soil, and dust. And it is shockingly common in cosmetics, especially in lipstick. Avoiding the lead in cosmetics is within our power, but breathing it in 17,280 times every day probably isn't—every breath contains a fresh dose of it.

Our bodies do not easily break lead down. Consequently, it accumulates in our blood, bone, and soft tissues where it causes problems with the nervous system, kidneys, liver, and other organs. Children are especially susceptible to lead toxicity, even at low doses. A small accumulation of lead in a child can cause central nervous system damage and result in slowed growth that can have a lifetime of consequences.

Even water contains toxins gathered from the air on its way down from the clouds to earth. Add to that the possible 127+ chemicals that the World Health Organization (WHO) identified in drinking water[3] and suddenly this element so critical to our survival seems more like a swamp than an oasis. We may filter our water at home, but as soon as we go out into the world we are subject to an aqua-onslaught of toxins.

Not to mention that water is the first or second listed ingredient in most Big Cosmo skincare products. *Unfiltered water. Water contaminated with environmental hazards as well as air polluted toxins. Drinking filtered water is great, but not if you are dousing your largest organ multiple times daily with it.* Big Cosmo uses unfiltered water as the primary ingredient because it is cheap—cheap and dirty, yet sounds so harmless. Water has no place in most skin care products. It contributes no nutrients—in fact, it actually removes nutrients as it evaporates from the skin leading to dehydrations and aging. *It's probably the best-kept dirty secret they keep—until now.*

Soil pollution travels from place to place as it is moved by air, water, or transport. Where it lands, it brings with it the contaminants previously dropped onto or buried in it.

Consider this example: Soil from below a factory smokestack is layered with contaminants that drop from the smokestack onto the ground. When that soil is blown and dispersed over miles during

3 http://www.who.int/water_sanitation_health/publications/2011/9789241548151_ch12.pdf?ua=1

a windstorm, it deposits those contaminants along its path. What happens in one portion of the world eventually finds its way to other parts. What we do to the environment comes back to haunt us in its destructive effects on our bodies.

The earth's ozone layer has been depleted over decades, allowing more ultraviolet rays from the sun to impact our health. The Union of Concerned Scientists predicts that within the next decade, higher ground-level ozone concentrations caused by global warming could cause about 1.4–2.8 million more cases of respiratory diseases, most of which will affect the most vulnerable—seniors and children—and add billions to our national healthcare costs.[4]

Most of us already know that being in the sun without skin protection is a recipe for disaster, so we slather on UV protective creams or lotions. But at what cost? Are we protecting our skin from UV rays while polluting our bloodstream with chemicals that cause metabolic disruption and a range of illnesses? Most sunscreens contain chemicals that disrupt the hormone system, are toxic to our reproductive system, or hinder normal development.

Just by being air-breathing, water-drinking mammals we are bombarded by chemicals outside of our control. I'm not trying to scare you, but I do want to bring the gravity of the situation to your attention. After reading this book, I hope you'll read the labels on all commercial products and become informed about the many harmful ingredients they contain.

But this book is not about the uncontrollable pollutants in the air, water, soil, and light. It's about our power to limit our exposure—and that of our families—in at least one important area: our skincare.

---

4 http://www.ucsusa.org/publications/ask/2011/ozone-depletion.html

HOW WE WORK
Our Amazing Skin

Earlier, I reminded you that our skin is the largest organ of the body. Did you know it covers a surface area of roughly six feet and can contribute to approximately 16 percent of your total body weight? It's constantly changing—replenishing itself at a rate of about 30,000–40,000 cells a minute. This means that each year you lose and regenerate about nine pounds (4.1 kilograms) of skin.[5]

The skin contains three layers—epidermis, dermis, and subcutaneous. Each layer performs specific functions to help cover and protect your body, regulate body temperature, and provide your sense of touch.

When we look at our skin we see the *epidermis*. As any facial scrub lover knows, the epidermis is constantly sloughing off dead cells, which is exactly what facial scrubs remove. The epidermis is what makes the skin our first barrier to infection. It also regulates how much water is released so we don't walk around all shriveled up from dehydration. And, it is our first vehicle of absorption when we put on lotions or creams. It is why some medications are transdermal—applied on the skin for rapid absorption and quick effects.

Below it is the *dermis,* where we find the nerve endings, blood vessels, hair follicles, oil, and sweat glands. It also contains collagen and elastic fibers—proteins that keep skin firm and strong. And the dermis helps cushion the body from stress and strain.

Finally, there's the *subcutaneous* layer—also called the *hypodermis*—which is made up mostly of fat. Here is where the greatest chemical impact from skincare products lies because fat is where

---

5 http://kidshealth.org/kid/htbw/skin.html

toxins and chemicals end up when they cannot be eliminated by the body. Toxins can live in fat cells for many years, and can cause strange symptoms when they are suddenly eliminated through detox or weight loss.

The way fat harbors toxins is also why detox can take much longer than expected. To really detox, you must find a way to get those toxins and chemicals out of fat storage, and this is usually a gradual process over time that can have a variety of manifestations.

Our amazing skin is a workhorse. It has so many functions, all of which are vital to daily health. Let's look at them:

Waterproofing:

The epidermis contains a layer of cells called *stratum corneum*, which are very tightly packed cells meant to protect against absorption of substances. This is the reason your body doesn't suck up all the water when you jump into the swimming pool. Without the mighty epidermis you would swell with water weight gain every time you took a shower, no matter what time of the month it is.

Evaporation:

The epidermis provides a relatively dry and semi-impermeable barrier to reduce fluid loss and dehydration.

Protection:

When the epidermis is healthy it protects the body from bacteria, viruses, infections, and other unwanted substances. Langerhans cells in the epidermis are part of our adaptive immune system that protects us from infection. The natural layer of oil that is part of our skin's outer layer is our first barrier of protection, but many chemicals and toxins in skincare products actually strip away this natural oil. I touch on this in Chapter Nine (the men's chapter that many women may want to read as well), but it is worth mentioning here, too.

Harsh chemicals (sodium lauryl sulfate and triclosan, among others) in soaps, conditioners, body washes, and face washes strip away the layer of protective oils your skin creates. Along with this protective layer goes your body's first line of defense.

Sebum, the oil from your sebaceous glands, contains medium-chain triglycerides (MCTs) just like those found in coconut oil (a great reason to put coconut oil on your skin). Protective bacteria live on the surface of your skin. There is actually more bacteria that live on the surface of your skin than in your body. These lipophilic microbes (natural surface bacteria) actually consume the glycerol portion of the MCT and leave behind fatty acids. Fatty acids (called medium-chain fatty acids or MCFAs) are protective by nature because they naturally kill pathogenic bacteria, viruses, and fungi.

The washes from my Primal Life Organics skincare line cleanse the surface of your skin but leave this protective layer intact—your skin will not have that dry, tight feeling AND your first line of defense remains intact because you get to keep your MCFAs! This is also a protective feature for cuts, rashes, irritations, lacerations, ulcerations or any open skin lesion that could become infected. Washing with a harsh soap washes away your first line of defense against that wound becoming contaminated and infected. Leave your natural defenses intact, and your impaired skin has a better chance of healing quickly.

Sense of touch:
Nerve endings in the dermis give you your fifth sense, also referred to as somatosensory or haptic perception. They respond to heat and cold, touch and pressure, vibration, and tissue injury. Without this, we wouldn't know if we stepped on glass or put our hand on a hot surface.

Thermoregulation:

The dermis maintains our body temperature through the production of sweat and control of evaporation—a process known as insensible perspiration. Eccrine (sweat) glands in the dermis secrete sweat, which then evaporates on the surface of the skin. Sweat glands and dilated blood vessels aid heat loss when we're too hot, and constricted vessels greatly reduce the dermis' blood flow to conserve heat when we get cold. Sweating is a natural process you want to allow to happen. Sweat contains cellular waste products and toxins produced within your body. Sweat is a natural, protective mechanism of the body to get rid of these toxins. Using antiperspirants that prohibit this process (prevent sweating) not only prevent thermoregulation, but cause a build up of cellular waste and toxins within the body.

Storage and synthesis:

Subcutaneous skin cells act as a storage center for lipids (fats) and water. As we saw above, chemicals and toxins can sit contentedly in the fat cells for years, slowly contaminating the body and causing a wide array of life-long health issues.

Our skin is strong and powerful, but it is responsive to its environment, especially a polluted one. And it is easily suffocated by layers of toxins. Polluted skin can be compared to living with a cold 24/7, 365 days a year. Cells can't get oxygen, and nutrients cannot be absorbed or utilized. Before long, the skin is so congested it cannot function, and becomes stressed. Toxins accumulate and symptoms like acne, rosacea, rashes, bumps, and other irritations begin to appear.

I am living proof that eliminating toxic skincare products can change long-standing issues. I lived with oily skin and acne for years. When I first created my own toxin-free moisturizer, those problems disappeared.

HOW WE WORK
Our Amazing Endocrine System

We may never think of it, but the endocrine system influences almost every cell, organ, and function of our bodies. It is in charge of body processes that happen slowly, like the rise and fall of hormone levels.

The endocrine system is the collection of cells, glands, and tissues that secrete hormones directly into the bloodstream. Some are transported along nerve tracts to control physiological and behavioral activities. It may be powerful, but our endocrine system is also delicate and easily affected.

Producing and regulating hormones is a complicated task that creates slow results over time. Faster processes like breathing and body movement are controlled by the nervous system. Although the nervous and endocrine systems are separate, they often work together.

Because most commercial chemicals negatively affect the endocrine system, the nurse in me wants to make sure you understand what the heck it is. Here are the components of our complex endocrine system:

1. Adrenal glands
2. Hypothalamus
3. Intestines
4. Kidneys
5. Parathyroid for calcium regulation
6. Pineal body

7. Pituitary gland
8. Reproductive organs (ovaries, testes, uterus, and placenta when pregnant)
9. Thyroid

Hormones and glands are the foundation of the endocrine system. Hormones are the body's chemical messengers—they transfer information and instructions from one set of cells to another. Many different hormones move through the bloodstream, but each type is designed to affect only certain cells.

A gland is a group of cells that produces and secretes organic chemicals. Glands select and remove materials from the blood, process them, and secrete the finished chemical product for use somewhere in the body. Endocrine glands release more than twenty major hormones directly into the bloodstream for transport to various cells.

Endocrine disruptors (EDs) or endocrine disrupting compounds (EDCs) are substances that interfere with the production of hormones by either inhibiting or exaggerating it. You may see them listed as "hormonally active agents" or "xenohormones."

Many laboratory studies have demonstrated the harmful biological effects of EDs on animals. Even in doses lower than those used in laboratory experiments, they have similar effects on humans.[6] The Endocrine Society states that EDs and EDCs affect reproduction, breast development and cancer, prostate cancer, neuro-endocrinology, metabolism and obesity, and cardiovascular endocrinology.[7]

The most critical time of hormonal influence is during early cell formation in pregnancy, when a hormone imbalance can have profound effects.

---

6 http://www.who.int/ipcs/publications/new_issues/endocrine_disruptors/en/
7 http://press.endocrine.org/doi/abs/10.1210/er.2009-0002

Such disruptions have the potential to cause cancerous tumors, birth defects, and developmental disorders. Deformed bodies—including limbs—can result from poorly regulated hormones. The sad evidence of this is the number of birth defects of babies born to mothers in the 1960–70s who took diethylstilbestrol (aka thalidomide) for morning sickness and nausea. Many of these babies had truncated, ill-formed, or missing arms.

One powerful ED is the phthalate group of chemicals, used as softening agents in everything from nail products to personal care to children's toys. Why is this chemical included in any product—much less in children's products—when it is known to cause neurological damage and development defects, changes in the testes and prostate, reduce sperm count, and can also affect fetal development?

Learning disabilities, cognitive and brain problems, and severe attention deficit disorder can be caused by malfunction of the endocrine system. Does this make you (like me) question whether skyrocketing rates of autism and ADHD could be caused by environmental, skincare, and dietary toxins?

Endocrine disruption produces masculinized effects in females and feminized effects in males. In Chapter Nine, we will talk further about decreased male fertility, deformed sperm, and increased rates of breast cancer in males. The American Cancer Society projects that in 2014 there will be about 2,360 new cases of invasive breast cancer diagnosed, and about 430 men will die from breast cancer.[8]

Endocrine disrupting compounds in the environment have been linked to reproductive problems and infertility in wildlife. Happily, an upsurge in fertility and a reduction of health problems

---

8 http://www.cancer.org/cancer/breastcancerinmen/detailedguide/breast-cancer-in-men-key-statistics

in some wildlife populations have been linked to bans and restricted use of EDCs in the wild. We can look at this hopeful example as we consider what happens in our bodies when we choose to eliminate chemicals from our skincare products and our diets.

Are you surprised to realize that the scientific community is still in debate about the negative effects of EDs, the dosage at which they are safe, and the long-term effects of prenatal exposure to them? Some groups demand that all EDs be immediately removed from the market, but some scientists and regulators want further studies, despite the growing mountain of evidence against their use.

In a paper for Tufts University, researchers reported many startling conclusions: The exposure necessary for "profound physiological effects" is much lower than we thought; endocrine disruptors are more widely found than previously assumed; humans are exposed to these chemicals at nearly every turn in household and industrial products. They affect every hormonal system. And intra-utero exposure can create effects that may not be seen until adulthood.[9]

Wow! It is shocking to think of all the chemicals we come in contact with every day and the range of consequences that they carry. Studies show that the average woman applies more than 500 chemicals to her body during her daily beauty routine. Environmental Working Group (EWG) and The Campaign for Safe Cosmetics is a great resource for finding products and their toxic count. I highly suggest looking into this resource when searching for the best alternatives!

Is there really a good reason to add more fuel to the fire, or should I say, chemicals to the body? Everything we apply to our skin is absorbed and affects our well being from the outside, in.

Not only do commercial chemicals cause damage to our insides, they promote aging on both the inside and outside of the body.

---

9 http://www.tufts.edu/~skrimsky/PDF/neurotoxicology.PDF

Dehydrated, congested cells cannot perform properly. Big Cosmo's chemical brew is anything but anti-aging and healthy. They never include warnings on their labels and the less you know, the better off they are. They entice you with fancy chemicals, real ingredients and "organic" labeling, however, they don't disclose how harmful the fillers they put in their products really are. Any positive effect their "good" ingredients may have is surely overpowered by the abundance of water, chemicals and toxins. Their labels really should include this: *Warning: this product may make you fat, sick and forgetful.* There's more...

HOW WE WORK
What about the rest of the body?

Understanding how endocrine disruptors affect the endocrine system is extremely important, but did you know that *these chemicals affect your entire body?*

Chemicals can cause cell mutations. As cells reproduce, they replicate the mother cell. A mutated cell will most likely form another mutated cell, and many of these are precursors to cancer cells. After all, cancer is simply an overgrowth of mutated cells.

Chemicals also are irritants that can cause inflammation. Strong evidence suggests that almost all disease stems from an inflammatory process. Cardiac disease, pancreatic disease (diabetes), liver disease, bowel disorders, respiratory disease (asthma, Chronic Obstructive Pulmonary Disease), and kidney disease can all be linked to the inflammatory process.

Your brain cannot hide from these chemicals either. Remember that these chemicals love fat, and your brain contains a large percentage of fat, so these chemicals will easily target it. Symptoms include attention deficit, memory loss, confusion, and difficulty concentrating. One study linked Alzheimer's disease to the aluminum found in commercial deodorant.

Chemicals and toxins also destroy the immune system. Our immune system is our defense mechanism against poisons entering the body. The liver is our main organ of detoxification, and a fully functional liver supports our immune system. Toxins cause free radicals that destroy the cells of the body and bind to cytokines (immune system information pathways), damaging them and resulting in weakened immune system responses.

However, the damage is not just directly from the chemical or toxin. Once inside the body, most chemicals or toxins are broken down, or produce subsequent toxins. Toxins produced by petrochemicals (petroleum), phthalates, parabens, and other endocrine disruptors are xenoestrogens, meaning they mimic estrogen in the body and contribute to hormone imbalance, with subsequent immune suppression.

A weakened immune system compromises our entire being, making us susceptible to infection, inflammation (remember cardiac disease is an inflammatory disease), allergies, asthma, autoimmune disorders like rheumatoid arthritis, inflammatory bowel disease (IBD), lupus, multiple sclerosis, type 1 diabetes, Guillain-Barré syndrome, eczema, and allergic rhinitis.

Finally, your skin itself is not immune to these chemicals. Most chemicals are skin irritants and can cause numerous skin conditions. Have you ever thought that your acne, rosacea, rashes, or irritations could be *caused* by your skincare? The truth is, yes—the chemicals found in commercial skincare products can cause all of these issues and more. In fact, most of the chemicals added to commercial skincare are so toxic and caustic to the skin that lab personnel are required to wear protective gear while handling them.

Furthermore, these chemicals must be disposed of carefully because they are also toxic to the environment. Some are so potent and deadly they have to be buried deep within the ground.

Without exaggeration, your commercial skincare is making you fat, sick, and forgetful, without you being aware—until NOW!

LABELS
Know What You're Reading

"Read the label." You've heard that advice a thousand times. And even though you trust the words "natural" and "organic," maybe you occasionally check out that long list of increasingly mysterious ingredients in your favorite cleanser, moisturizer, shaving cream, or lipstick. Unfortunately, labels can be misleading and create a false sense of security.

What does "natural" mean in the world of the cosmetic industry? If the list of ingredients is unpronounceable, which part is natural?

The real and frightening issue behind the labeling deception in skincare is that chemicals exist in every type of commercial body care product, even the ones labeled "natural." Most of us use multiple products every single day! That means we take a chemical bath every time we apply commercial products to our skin.

Some natural or organic products are anything but that. Often, they contain only a few truly natural or organic ingredients. Sure, there may be a few ingredients that fit the definition, but your favorite product likely contains various other components that are harmful to the body as well as to the environment.

When I discovered that EVERYTHING I was putting on my skin contained chemicals... I was mortified. It was fairly easy to give up most of my products knowing they were doing more harm than good… but makeup?! That was not easy!! Especially since my complexion was less than attractive at the time. My skin was extremely oily, my forehead was infested with acne bumps, I was blotchy and had old acne scars.

However, makeup contains some of the most harmful ingredients. And once we apply it, it just sits there for the remainder of our day—clogging our pores, disrupting our hormones and altering our cells.

Makeup containing inorganic pigments like mica, zinc oxide, and iron oxide is hugely popular and often touted as a "natural alternative" to conventional products. Though these minerals do come from the ground, they have to go through chemical purification processes before they can be included in cosmetics, and they carry those chemicals into the "natural" skincare products.

Another controversy surrounding minerals in makeup involves the use of ultra-fine—nano-sized—particles. Once inside the body, all organs (including the brain) and tissues are open for entry by these miniscule particles. But no one knows for sure to what extent these particles affect our cells in the long term.

What's more, some makeup brands use potentially harmful minerals like talc, aluminum, and bismuth oxychloride (a by-product of lead and ore refining that can scratch the surface of the skin and cause skin irritation).

The ingredients that make up any manufactured product are listed in order of importance on the label, i.e., the percentage they compose of the product. The first ingredient listed represents the largest percentage of the mixture; the second is the next most predominant, etc.

But the reality is that many products marketed as "natural" are misnomers because they may contain only 15 percent natural components. That leaves 85 percent that are unnatural and can be extremely harmful to your body.

Many "natural" products contain emulsifiers, preservatives, and fragrances. These can cause endocrine disruption, cancer, DNA damage, as well as a plethora of other bodily dysfunctions that sneak up over time.

It's difficult to correlate forgetfulness with your deodorant. But what do most commercial deodorants contain? Aluminum—in the form of aluminum chlorohydrate.

Aluminum chlorohydrate in commercial deodorants inhibits sweat by plugging up sweat glands. *This prevents their detoxifying function: expelling chemicals and toxins.* Aluminum chlorohydrate is easily absorbed through the skin and has, in the only reported trial to date, been linked with higher risks of Alzheimer's disease.

When aluminum blocks sweat from being released, these toxins are stuck in the body and easily migrate to other nearby tissues and organs. Toxins and chemicals *seek out* fatty tissue, and what's the closest fatty organ to your armpit? Your brain.

Another very common ingredient in commercial skincare products is water. Humans require water, so what could possibly be wrong with it being a main ingredient in your skincare product? In fact, many commercial skincare products, even the natural ones, list water as the first ingredient. So who cares if your product is mostly water?

Water may be the perfect liquid for your insides, but your outsides feel differently. It might just be where all destructive effects truly begin.

Don't get me wrong; hydrating the skin is a good thing. However, most of the water in your skincare (lotion, cream, balm) evaporates before the skin absorbs it. As water evaporates, it takes with it many of the skin's natural oils. This actually makes your skin *lose* moisture and contributes to dryness.

Further, if water is the first ingredient on the label, it is likely that 75–95 percent of what's in the tube is simply water. Remember, the water Big Cosmo is putting in your skin care is *not filtered* and contains pollutants from the air as well and environmental and industrial. If that product contains any oils (and most natural products do), an emulsifier is necessary to make the water and oil mix and not separate. Most common emulsifiers in skincare include cetyl alcohol and sorbitan oleate, stearyl alcohol, stearic acid and triethanolamine.

Sodium laureth sulfate (SLS) is a common emulsifier used in products that foam (shampoo, detergents, bubble bath, etc.) as well as in toothpaste. If you check out the chart at the end of the chapter, you'll see that SLS promotes the formation of a group of carcinogenic compounds called nitrosamines. SLS also damages the epidermis and causes skin irritation. Children who soak in a tub of bubble bath, for instance, are especially vulnerable to urinary infections caused by SLS.

If an emulsifier is present, preservatives are *always* included to keep the product from spoiling, and parabens are the most common preservative. Parabens promote the production of estrogen and are increasingly linked to early puberty in girls. Naturally occurring parabens are found in some foods that are metabolized in the body (by the liver), lessening their estrogen-production effects.

One of the most common preservatives is the group of synthetic parabens. Unfortunately, synthetic parabens cannot be metabolized like naturally occurring ones. They increase estrogen production, disrupt hormone functions, and cause DNA damage.

Parabens are directly linked to breast cancer and cause negative reproductive effects in both females and males. Because of the vast array of cosmetics women use, it is estimated that women absorb about 50mg of synthetic parabens every day. And here's a dose of irony: parabens in skincare products *promote skin aging*.

Here are some examples of personal skincare products, which consist primarily of water:

Bath foam	Mascara
Conditioner	Mouthwash
Creams, moisturizers	Nail polishes (some)
Foundation	Self-tanning lotion
Hair gel	Shampoo
Hair spray	Shaving foam or lotion
Liquid eyeliner	Toothpaste
Makeup remover	

Not every product included here will list water as the first or second ingredient, but the majority of commercial products will. Many expensive anti-aging serums are 70 percent water, and shampoos can be as much as 90 percent.

So, if water, emulsifier, and preservatives are part of the product, that means that the rest of the ingredients are the active ingredients—the reason you bought the product in the first place. For most commercial products, if you take out the water, emulsifier, and fillers, the active ingredients will only be between 2 to 25 percent! Clearly, what you are buying is filler, not active ingredients. Fillers are cheap, ineffective and most likely harmful to your body, but they make Big Cosmo money!

Chemicals, dyes, fragrances, and other artificial ingredients in skin care and cosmetics are irritating to the skin. Often, they dehydrate skin cells. This can lead to health issues as well as premature aging.

Worse, some ingredients are toxic to multiple body systems and can cause disruption to organ function, such as thyroid malfunction. A few are known carcinogens—things that can cause cancer.

Propylene glycol (PG) is commonly used as a thickener, a softener, and to enhance penetration/absorption.

It is also a basic component in brake fluid, hydraulic fluid, floor wax, and paint. It is the main ingredient in anti-freeze. My car's mechanical needs and my biological needs are vastly different, but the cosmetic industry apparently doesn't see it that way.

The range of products intended for humans but containing PG is astounding—most cosmetics (especially lipstick and liquid foundation), deodorants, moisturizers, suntan lotions, baby wipes, and even ice cream.

PG is linked to a host of endocrine issues: DNA and cell deformation, kidney and liver diseases, inhibited cell growth, and generalized system toxicity. To that list of biological disruption add the fact that during production PG is easily contaminated with the cancer-causing chemical, dioxane.

Ingredients like those in commercial deodorants are increasingly found in the lumps and tumors of breast tissue. And, although the American Cancer Society reports that women still account for 99 percent of breast cancer diagnoses in the United States—and men are about 100 times less likely than women to get it—breast cancer in men is on the rise. In the past three years, cases of breast cancer in men have increased by 13.7 percent (compared to a 12.1 percent increase in women).

If men's breast tissue is now being affected by something that is typically a woman's disease, imagine what that toxic load is doing to their prostates. Hormone disruption has been linked with prostate cancer as well as male infertility.

Today we know of around 3,100 stock chemical ingredients that make up fragrance alone. If you see fragrance listed on your skincare product—buyer beware! Fragrance is considered a trade secret, meaning the ingredients do not need to be disclosed. Most chemicals that make up fragrances are neurotoxins. The list below is only the tip of the chemical iceberg!

Toxic overload accumulates over time. It can begin in utero and continue throughout our lives. Toxins affect our kidneys, liver, thyroid, bowels, endocrine system, skin, and even our brain. Remember that aluminum-filled deodorant? No? You might want to check your risk for Alzheimer's disease! These toxins and chemicals can affect us in myriad subtle ways that aren't evident until they are a serious problem.

These are the not-so-beautiful secrets Big Cosmo hides. They don't want you to discover the truth behind their lies. They don't want you to question their ingredient lists, intentions or standards. Don't play skincare roulette! It's just not worth it. Children are even more susceptible to these chemicals because they have a higher body fat percentage and more rapid absorption rate. And babies have immature neurologic and immune systems—two crucial systems directly affected by the chemicals in commercial skincare.

I've included a chart of Big Cosmo's Dirty Secrets: Chemicals commonly found in most skincare at the end of this chapter. Please note that *thousands* of chemicals are disclosed as part of modern life, but it is impossible to know how many are undisclosed. This is just a very short list of the most common.

The hidden, long-term effects of toxic chemicals in our bodies was my main concern when I gave serious attention to how many chemicals in both commercial and natural products assault our biological balance at every turn.

The good news was that, in contrast, natural, real-food skin care products clean and nourish us from our outside skin to our deepest inside cells. I knew there had to be a way to have beauty and health, too. It shouldn't have to be a trade-off.

Creating my own skincare from real food Primal Life Organics was my answer to that dilemma. Getting back to the basics. Revealing the Great Skin Lies and Beauty's Dirty Secret. Removing the lab and bringing in the dirt. Anti-aging and health is more of a lifestyle and mindset than chemical created in a lab. Convert your thinking from skincare to skin-food and something happens! Real. Skin. Food. Nourishes. Protects. Heals.

Ditching the chemicals becomes easier when you know what they are doing to your body. It's the first step to Super Power your skin. Discover what Big Cosmo is hiding from you- and discover what your skin can be like if not under-the-chemical-influence. Detoxing from a chemical-laden life to a nutrient-dense one is the second step in Super Powering your skin!

When I bought this item a few months ago, I was desperate for change for my skin. Over time using the Bare Package, my skin became firmer, clearer, and softer. The cleanser washes off without being harsh or stripping my skin's natural oils. The moisturizer feels amazing at the end of the day and gives my skin a glow. It's amazing! Thank you PLO!

—Libby

Big Cosmo's Dirty Secrets
Chemicals Commonly Found in
Commercial Skincare Products

Chemical	Use	Effects	Found In
PARABENS Naturally occur in some foods and are metabolized in the body, mitigating much of their estrogenic effects. **Synthetic parabens** found in cosmetics and absorbed into body through the skin are *not* metabolized, therefore have much more potent estrogenic effects.	**Preservative**	• Endocrine disruptor • Disrupt hormone function • Linked to breast cancer • Linked to negative reproductive effects in females and males • Causes skin aging • Causes DNA damage It is estimated that women absorb about 50 mg. of parabens *daily.*	• Moisturizers • Shampoos and conditioners • Many types of makeup

Chemical	Use	Effects	Found In
PHTHALATES	**Softeners**	• Endocrine disruptors • Interferes with hormone function • Reproductive damage—may affect fertility • May affect fetus • Neurological damage • Promote genetic mutation ability of other chemicals • Developmental defects • Testes and prostate changes • Reduced sperm counts • Easily absorbed through skin	• Nail products • Personal care products • Cosmetics • Children's toys
ACRYLAMIDE	**Binder** **Film former** **Thickener**	• Link to mammary tumors • Increases infertility • Increases neurological problems	• Face creams
DIETHANOL- **AMINE** **(DEA)**	**Wetting agent** **Foaming agent** **pH adjuster** (counteracts acidity of other ingredients)	• Forms potent carcinogen • (nitrosodietha-nolamine NDEA) when combined with other cosmetic chemicals • Linked to stomach, esophagus, liver and bladder cancers	• Personal care (soaps, cleansers, shampoo) • Laundry detergent • Cleaning products

Chemical	Use	Effects	Found In
PETROLATUM (Mineral Oils & Paraffin)	**Base**	• Hormone disruptor • Can slow cellular development • Promotes aging • Suspected carcinogen • Coats skin & clogs pores • Creates build-up of toxin	• Creams • Baby rash ointment • Personal care products
SODIUM LAURETH SULFATE (SLS) Originally developed as a pesticide and aggressive chemical cleaner for heavy oil stains in garages and car washes Manufacture of SLS creates ethoxylation which contains the carcinogen, dioxane	**Detergent Dispersant Emulsifier Foaming agent Wetting agent**	• Forms nitrosamines (carcinogenic compound) when combined with other chemicals • Damages outer layer of skin • Causes skin irritation (This property is sometimes promoted in order to increase the penetration of other components of the cosmetic.) • Urinary infections (especially in children from soaking in the tub)	• Toothpaste • Shampoo • Face and body cleansers • Laundry • Household cleaning • Bubble bath

Chemical	Use	Effects	Found In
PROPLENE GLYCOL (PG) **This IS anti-freeze!** Also found in brake and hydraulic fluid, floor wax, and paints Petroleum-based, produced as side product from petroleum refining	**Thickener Solvent Softener Moisture-carrier** **Penetration enhancer** (expands skin permeability & increases absorption)	• Linked to kidney and liver disease • Easily contaminated with the carcinogen, dioxane • Possible genetic and cell deformation • Possible inhibitor of cell growth • Skin irritation, contact dermatitis, rashes, dry skin • Systemic toxicity	• Cosmetics • Shampoo & conditioners • Deodorant • Liquid foundation • Spray deodorant • Moisturizers • Lipsticks • Suntan lotions • Baby wipes • Ice cream!
PHENOL (CARBOLIC ACID) Petroleum product Banned in Canadian cosmetics	**Aromatic compound**	• Corrosive to eyes, skin, respiratory tract • Causes lung edema • Harmful to central nervous system and heart • Causes dysrhythmia, seizures, coma • May affect kidneys • Possibly toxic to non-reproductive organs	• Skin lotion
PETROLEUM (Mineral oil)	**Moisturizer**	• Carcinogen • Skin irritant • Allergen	• Face and body moisturizers • Hair products

Chemical	Use	Effects	Found In
DIOXANE 1,4 Not required to be listed on product labels because it is a contaminant created during manufacturing	**Foaming agent**	• Linked to cancer • Derived from ethylene oxide, a known breast carcinogen	• Shampoo • Baby shampoo • Bubble bath • Body wash • Liquid soap • Detergent
FRAGRANCE Over 3,000 chemicals are used to create different scents ***Be aware:** Fragrance recipes are considered trade secrets so manufacturers are not required to disclose fragrance chemicals in the list of ingredients	**Scent** Even "fragrance-free" or "unscented" products may have fragrance ingredients	• Neurotoxins • Carcinogens • Loss of muscle control • Brain damage • Headaches • Memory loss • Speech problems • Hearing problems • Vision problems • Musk ketone accumulates in breast milk and fatty tissues	• Perfume • Cologne • Deodorant • Nearly every type of personal care product • Laundry detergents • Softeners • Cleaning products
FORMALDEHYDE Highly toxic to all humans and animals, no matter how it's ingested	**Preservative**	• Known carcinogen • Toxic to immune system • Toxic to respiratory tract • Skin irritant • Eye irritant • Injurious to upper gastrointestinal tract	• Nail polish • Body lotion • Body wash • Cleansers • Shampoo & conditioners • Styling gel • Sunscreen • Makeup

Chemical	Use	Effects	Found In
TALCUM POWDER Helps products stick to the skin and promotes translucency	**Absorbent Lubricant**	• May contain asbestos (carcinogen) • Possible link to ovarian cancer • Link to inflammatory lung disorders including cancer • Link to adrenal cancers	• Eye shadow • Baby powder • Feminine hygiene products
SILICONES SILOXANES: Cyclotetrasiloxane, Cyclopentasiloxane, Cyclohexasiloxane and Cyclomethicone	**Softener Smoothening agent Moisturizer Lubricant Drying agent**	• Endocrine disruptor • Fertility inhibitor • Carcinogen • Immune system disruptor	• Skin and hair products • Makeup (foundation, blush, eye shadow, eye liners, lipstick)
TRICLOSAN	**Antibacterial agent**	• Possible endocrine disruptor • Affects testosterone & sperm count • Affects estrogen levels (early-onset puberty)	• Soap • Toothpaste • Skin care products • Plastics • Fabrics

CHAPTER FIVE

Detox: The Super Power Boot Camp

"Detox"—the word evokes images of wayward people with destructive drug or alcohol habits creating poisonous levels of toxins that must be eliminated before their bodies can function normally again. Commercial skincare products cause a chemical poisoning that is equally toxic, but few people talk about where that toxicity comes from or how to eliminate it.

Detoxifying your skin and body is the second step in creating Super Power skin. Super Power skin is radiant and glowing because the cells are receiving the nutrients they need to manage waste, utilize oxygen and nutrients, and replicate healthy cells. Super Power your skin and you will look younger, have more tone and elasticity and exhibit a radiant glow. The process of detoxifying is your skin's *Super Power Boot Camp. What is detox and how will it effect you?*

Detox—detoxification—is what we do to purge ourselves of things that are bad for us. Toxins can be anything—poisons we put into our bodies, drug or alcohol addictions that twist and control our lives, or relationships that destroy our psyches.

Most people have had the experience of trying to eliminate a negative force from their lives to free themselves of its debilitating effects. Sometimes we're successful and sometimes we're not, but in the process we learn a great deal about ourselves— we identify our strengths and weaknesses and we discover which tools work best.

Drugs and alcohol eventually cause obvious physical changes, make others reluctant to be with us, or create complex problems that demand elaborate and often expensive solutions. They affect our vitality, induce skin problems like lesions, or attack our nerves so that we cannot rest enough to keep our immune system functional. They invade our brains by crossing the blood-brain barrier and impair judgment, both while we're under the influence and when we're sober. The resulting laundry list of health problems is a story unto itself.

But what happens when we are exposed to toxins via the chemicals we unknowingly put into our body through commercial skincare? In a subtle and long-term way, our vitality is lessened, skin problems develop, and our endocrine system cannot help our immune system keep us healthy. Chemicals and toxins from skincare also cross the blood-brain barrier and invade our brains. We have already mentioned the possible link between the aluminum in commercial deodorant and Alzheimer's disease. There's a world of social difference between drug and alcohol poisoning and commercial skincare poisoning, but they look pretty much the same to our endocrine, neurologic, metabolic, reproductive, and immune systems.

Commercial skincare has effectively put our skin in a chemical coma. Altering the way the cells function and ultimately destroying our innate natural skin story. Just like a drug, I was once addicted to commercial skincare. I spent thousands of dollars purchasing skincare that promised RESULTS such as; anti-aging, clear skin, less wrinkles, and even skin tone. Did I ever see any results? NO. Did I go back for more? YES. Why? I wanted to believe Big Cosmo was selling the same "miracle cream" that they had advertised so well… and my skin was in a trance.

The rapidly growing movement of people living (and eating) the Paleo way acknowledges that curbing everyday environmental toxins is beyond an individual's control, but they still want to know the consequences of mega doses of daily toxin exposure. They use their findings to seek natural, toxin-free alternatives. They begin with diet then incorporate as many healthy alternatives to normal commercial products as they can. They detoxify their environments, food sources, and skincare products in order to provide their bodies with sustainable nutrients.

By now you already know how important your endocrine system is for feeling and looking your best. You already know it underlies the well-being of all of your body's systems. And you know that excessive amounts of chemicals in commercially produced skincare products contribute to a myriad of problems that can make you or your child sluggish, unfocused, and overweight. You know absorption of these chemicals can lead to cancers, birth defects, developmental issues, or premature aging. Chemicals = toxins. Toxins = disease.

A healthy body quietly does a lot of detoxification every day. This natural function is triggered whenever a substance—good or bad—enters the body. Under most circumstances, constant vigilance by our immune system assures we maintain a natural balance that allows all our bio-systems to do their jobs. But toxins can suppress our natural responses and immune system.

A constant, daily barrage of poisonous substances can overwhelm even the healthiest of bodies. And the longer one is exposed to a substance, the longer it will take to detox from it. Of course, the opposite is also true: The shorter the exposure, the shorter the detoxification.

Those toxic substances are attracted to and easily stored in fat tissue and resist being broken down in water. The longer one is exposed to a toxin, the higher the level of that substance in fat/adipose tissue. And the more fat tissue, the more toxins can land in it, where they can happily stay for years.

Toxins are not stored only in our fat tissue, though. They can be stored in organ tissue—our brains, hearts, reproductive organs, livers, kidneys, pancreases, and skin.

It is easy to conclude that the more fat we store on our body, the more toxins we can harbor. The opposite can also be true. Someone who is lean will have less fat tissue available for these toxins to migrate into, meaning the liver will directly metabolize more toxins. For this reason, controlling our weight and BMI (body mass index) are clearly more important to health than we sometimes realize. The leaner we are, the fewer fat cells we have to store toxins. Period.

Eliminating stored toxins is difficult and requires a period of detoxification. The length of that period is dependent on numerous factors: how much has been stored, water intake and hydration levels, health issues, diet and skincare intake, and the functionality of your liver, skin, lungs, kidneys, and bowels. Your liver is primarily responsible for breaking down chemicals into water-soluble formulations that your kidney can easily remove through your urine. However, detoxification is multifaceted, and the skin, respiratory system, and bowels also do their fair share of breaking down and eliminating chemicals. In fact, congested skin (breakouts, rosacea, and other irritations) can be a sign of toxic infestation and your body's attempt to push those toxins out. Toxins invading the cells can also cause Irritable Bowel Syndrome (IBS), bloating, gas, and discomfort. Once chemicals enter our bodies, they alter us on the cellular level.

Without purification, toxins disrupt the cells' ability to function, and can cause mutations. Mutated cells will not function as the parent cells did—or they may not function at all. Disease is the result of cellular dysfunction. Diabetes, Alzheimer's disease, heart disease, and hypothyroidism lead to impaired livers, brains, hearts, and thyroid glands.

I witness detox every day in the hospital. Let me give you an example from my nursing experience to illustrate how the human body handles it. If you have ever experienced anesthesia, you will relate.

While you are under anesthesia you are given large doses of medication so a procedure can be performed without you being aware. But anesthesia is a foreign substance to your body—a chemical alteration of your normal. While anesthetized, some of the drug will be metabolized, some will invade your organs (your brain is the target organ and sleep is the desired outcome), but some of the drug will find its way into your fat tissue.

Over time, your liver metabolizes the drug. Once enough of the drug is metabolized, the level in your blood begins to fall lower than the level in your brain, and the drug will move from areas of higher concentration (brain and fat) to an area of lower concentration (the bloodstream). This is the law of distribution, which is followed by all drugs. Once the concentration falls below a certain threshold in your brain, you wake up.

However, you wake up slowly and feel groggy. Why? Because your fat tissue just tucked away a portion of the anesthesia. Over a period of time, the drug will redistribute and return to the bloodstream to be metabolized and eliminated. This process of elimination of a toxin—or detox—could take hours. Each person reacts individually, according to a wide variety of factors. Your reactions while detoxing may be different from someone else's.

The process—from introduction into the body, through the drug moving into your tissue and you feeling its effects, to its return to the bloodstream for metabolism and elimination—that's what detox is.

This is a very simple example of how the brain is influenced by a chemical to induce sleep and anesthesia, then how detox occurs as the brain partially awakens until the majority of the chemical is removed. Grogginess is the detox experience of the chemical leaving your brain.

Groggy is also how your cells function when under the influence of everyday chemicals and toxins in your body. Get rid of those chemicals and toxins, and your grogginess goes away.

Let's Talk Skincare!

When we use commercial skincare products, we are rubbing, scrubbing, and smoothing a multitude of chemical formulas into our bloodstream through our pores. If we use multiple products multiple times a day—*every* day—imagine the impact on our cells' functionality. It's not a huge stretch of the imagination to under-stand that this level of constant toxicity requires a significant detox period.

Because of the high levels of toxicity many of us experience, natural detox methods are important.

Natural methods are slower, but more thorough. When you detox the unwanted chemicals from your body, you will be sur-prised at how your body *really* feels and functions.

Changing your diet is crucial to detoxifying from the everyday barrage of our chemical-laden lives. It is one way by which you can take control of something you have the power to change. Changing your diet isn't complicated—just go organic and eat whole foods. Shop primarily from the outer aisles of the supermarket (where the produce is) and avoid processed foods of any kind, including mod-ern society's favorite poison: sugar. Sugar doesn't just cause rapid energy swings; it causes complex chemical reactions and produces the free radicals often responsible for cell death.

The switch to an organic diet can have immediate results— you will probably look and feel better. Eating organically gives your body a pure dose of easily digestible, nutrient-dense food. Every dose of goodness gives your body time and energy to remove stored toxins. By eating organically, you are giving your body a double dose of health: pure food and increased elimination.

While detoxifying, please remember to drink plenty of water every day. Drink a full glass upon waking to facilitate flushing out the toxins your body made while you rested.

During sleep, your body is still functioning. Healing and regen-eration occur during sleep. Overnight, the buildup of lactic acid and the waste products from bodily processes can result in a more sluggish awakening. A fresh glass of water will not only help remove those toxins, but will set you up for success to drink even more water throughout the day.

During detox, skip the coffee, soda (skip it anyway), and alcohol. All of these dehydrate you even more. Your goal is to rid your body of toxins—coffee, soda, and alcohol are part of that group.

Remember, you can sweat more if you have water to spare. Sweating is healthy because sweat contains toxins and your skin is a great organ for removal!

If you are interested in learning more about nutrition, diet, and health, look for a list of some of my favorite resources at the end of the book.

Adjustment and Detox: Your Super Power Skin

Let's say you've been on your new diet and skincare regime for a week. At first you feel so much better, have more energy, maybe people are commenting that your skin seems to "glow." But somewhere between week two and three of your organic-only diet, your glowing skin suddenly looks lifeless, congested, or broken out. Maybe you have a rash. And your newly discovered energy is nowhere to be seen.

What's going on? Aren't you supposed to be getting better, not worse?

I am here to tell you this: What you are experiencing is normal.

Remember all that fat and how it loves to store chemicals and toxins? Remember when I said natural processes take longer but are more thorough?

That is what is happening. Your body needed the prior weeks— the adjustment period—to find a way to seek out and remove toxins from your fat cells. Every time one cell empties its chemical contents into your bloodstream, it creates a small dose of toxicity, to which your body reacts.

The adjustment period is the skin's reaction to new products. If you have been using commercial products with alcohol or water as the first ingredients (like most commercial skincare products), your skin is in a constant state of dehydration. It cannot function properly so it adapts by increasing sebum production, a form of auto-regulation that fights against the drying effects of preservatives, fragrance, dyes, etc. Chemicals in commercial skincare products cause free radical production, which promotes premature aging, cellular mutation, and possibly even cancer.

The adjustment period is different from the detox period, although they happen simultaneously and can be difficult to distinguish.

Adjustment occurs every day. Changes to your lifestyle force you to adjust (consciously, unconsciously, physically, emotionally, rationally, and psychologically) and undergo a process of transformation. The same is true for skincare and purification.

During the detox period you may experience some of the following:

> You may feel dehydrated. During a detox you must drink *a lot* of water. Drinking purified water is more important than ever during a detox.

> Your energy may swing from high to low. Eat plenty of fresh fruits, vegetables, and fermented foods.

> You may experience diarrhea or constipation—two sides of the same coin.

> You may develop a rash, itching, dry skin, eczema, or psoriasis—congested skin cannot eliminate toxins well.

> Your immune system may be affected. You may be more susceptible to colds or viruses, experience flu symptoms, or observe a temporary allergic reaction. It may be more difficult to fight infections or heal.

> You may feel tired and need extra sleep. Listen to your body and take a nap or go to bed early. Sometimes your immune system is suppressed and will be weakened during its detox and adjustment.

> You may manifest something unusual because of your particular genetic makeup, diet, or the effects of the environment in which you live.

Don't be discouraged! Try to remember that if you quit in less than four weeks, you gave up way too early. Give yourself some time. You took years if not decades building this toxicity; it's not going to be gone in a month. Little by little, the toxins hidden deep in your cells will be released, until you no longer experience symptoms—because you are out of detox.

• • •

If the adjustment period and the actual detox period are so similar, how do you know which one you are experiencing? You might not. But generally, if your new symptoms occur within eight weeks of starting your new organic diet, you can assume it is detox. During the first four weeks, it could be one or the other, or even a combination of both.

Detox is like boot camp—it's not easy. You will experience unusual things. Your body will react, regress, respond, recharge and revamp. Your skin may show rebellion (acne, rashes, blotchiness, etc.) before it begins to glow. Hang in there, boot camp is not meant to be easy—it is meant to make you stronger. That's exactly what removing the chemicals will do for your skin and body. Detoxing from a chemical invasion will improve your health, however, it may not be an easy process. This process can take six months or longer.

Let's define the laws that govern your Detox Boot Camp that will leave you with Super Power Skin! The Laws of Concentration, Distribution and Redistribution define where and how much of a drug is in your body at a given time.

The **law of concentration** is the amount, or level, of a drug that is in your body. The levels vary from space to space. A drug may be more concentrated in your blood stream as opposed to your tissues. The **law of distribution** is simply where that drug is located. It is typically located in numerous places: fat tissue, blood stream, visceral tissue, organ tissue or bone tissue. The **law of redistribution** occurs as the levels change in relations to one another. A drug loves equilibrium and will always attempt to establish equilibrium. When the concentration drops in one area, the area of higher concentration will release (or give up) the drug to re-establish equilibrium between the tissues.

Putting it all together. Typically, your blood stream is the medium that sets the equilibrium because it is the highway that travels to all areas of concentration. When the concentration within the blood stream falls (via metabolism from the liver, lungs,

GI tract, bowels and skin; excretion from kidneys; or absorption into other tissues) your tissues will release more of the drug to re-establish equilibrium between the vascular system and tissues. This re-distribution occurs in opposite when the concentration in the tissue is less than the blood stream—this is how chemicals and toxins end up in your tissue in the first place. Your intake (either oral or via absorption through the skin) is greater than your tissue concentration. Since you lose the first pass through the liver when you absorb ingredients topically, your blood concentration may be higher than your tissue concentration. In an attempt to establish equilibrium—and prevent overdose in the blood, your body auto-regulates by storing the surplus amount in fatty tissue. This is also a self-protective mechanism of your body to help prevent large doses from reaching your brain. Remember, your brain is fat tissue and drugs are lipophilic (fat loving). If high concentrations reach your brain, they could migrate into the brain tissue and remain there until equilibrium is established—think concentration issues, ADD, Alzheimer's, drowsiness, mental confusion, etc.

When changing to a chemical free skincare routine, you enter Detox Boot Camp. During Detox Boot Camp, you are eliminating chemicals from entering your body. Therefore, your liver, kidneys, bowels, skin and lungs can now metabolize and excrete the levels within your blood—and your blood will be cleansed. As this clean blood travels throughout the body, it passes the tissues that store the surplus amounts of these chemicals and your tissues will release these toxins back into your blood, to re-establish equilibrium between the blood and tissue. If you continue to prevent chemical invasion, your equilibrium level will continue to drop until it is almost zero. This process can take a long time, and is dependent on hydration status, nutrition, health status, disease processes, environmental issues as well as activity level.

By arresting chemical invasion, eventually your tissues will detox most of the toxins back into your blood for metabolism into a water-soluble formula that can be excreted by your kidneys. Don't forget your skin also serves as a means for elimination and sometimes-congested skin can be related to toxic build up within the tissue of the skin. Congested skin can show its ugly face as acne, rosacea, peri-oral dermatitis, psoriasis and eczema. We will discuss these more in chapter seven. It's also not unusual for these conditions to occur or worsen during detox. Super Power skin happens after Boot Camp!

However, during detox you may feel better then worse then better, multiple times. Rest assured that your skin and body will heal, auto-regulate, and adjust to your new diet. Stay dedicated! Be grateful your body wants to work so hard to toss out toxins until your cells are filled with pure organic substances that optimize your health.

I have to insert here that the opposite is also true—if you fall off the organic wagon and resume a chemical-laden diet and use chemical-laden skincare, you will have an adjustment period too.

The media makes us expect everything fast—fast technology, fast medicine, fast talk. Speed sells, and it is worth millions. We've been sold the belief that faster is better because it benefits corporate profit margins, especially for pharmaceutical companies.

But the more we believe the speed hype, the less healthy we become. When you heal from the inside out, don't expect instant results. The laws of concentration–distribution–redistribution define how long it will take stored toxins to migrate out of the fat to be metabolized by the liver and eliminated by the kidneys via the urine, through the bowels via the feces, and by the lungs and skin. That's nature's safety measure.

I'm not sorry to tell you that undoing years of bad eating, using bad skincare products, or living a bad lifestyle doesn't happen overnight. It shouldn't. An overnight—or even fast—change would mean every cell would pour its toxins into your bloodstream at the same time and you could die from the chemical or emotional shock. Depending on your metabolism, prior use of commercial food or skincare products, and your water intake and activity level, a healthy detox should take about six months.

Thorough detoxing requires time and dedication, but you get something truly priceless in return: your health and more freedom from pain to live how you want to live, and longer.

Why don't people believe in detoxing from skincare and food pollution? They do not equate those things with drugs. But the chemicals that keep foods preserved for years or that make babies smell like bubblegum *are* drugs. And those drugs require a process to remove them from our bodies.

Levels of Detox:

A thorough detox occurs on several levels. Removing ALL toxins from your food and skincare will result in a nearly complete detox. Environmental factors beyond our control prevent us from achieving absolute detoxification. However, a body as free as possible from pesticides, ingested hormones, preservatives, and other chemicals will function more efficiently to remove the everyday pollution we can't avoid contacting.

When supply (of either a drug or a toxin) is completely discontinued, initial removal of the toxins is rapid, then tapers off until the remainder dwindles away over time.

If a drug or toxin is only decreased (not completely stopped), detox occurs until a new equilibrium is established.

The bad news is that since no one can achieve 100 percent removal of toxins from both food and skincare, the best we can all hope for is to live in a constant state of detox. If contamination is stopped, but then a small amount is re-introduced from time to time, a toxicity level of zero can never be established. This results in a person living in a constant state of intermittent detox caused by fluctuating doses of toxins. This up-and-down state can lead to skin conditions like acne, psoriasis, eczema, rashes, etc.

Give your body the fighting chance it needs to fully detox by incorporating both dietary and skincare options to heal your body from the inside out.

Here's the good news: If you fully detox your food and skincare products, an *occasional* (nobody's perfect) use or ingestion of them will not kill you or even set you back in your quest for excellent health. You've already given your body what it needs to function well, so your liver, for example, will efficiently do its job as the detoxifier and eliminator of toxins. The same goes for your detoxified kidneys, pancreas, skin, heart, lungs, and gut—because they're strong again, they can efficiently do their part to maintain your healthy balance.

Remember, your cells were the first to be damaged, which may have led to tissue damage, then organ damage, and finally system damage if overload occurred. Your body must first heal at the cellular level before you can see changes in your tissues; your tissues must heal first before you see changes in your organs; your cells, tissues and organs must all heal before your system will repair. Don't forget—your skin is an organ and will take some time to heal to the point where you see results.

Trading that pack of chemicals formed into cute bottles of strawberry-scented shower gel for all-natural skin food products rich in nutrients will keep your skin from being the first victim of toxins, and instead allow it to be your first line of defense.

I created *skin-food* to do just this. My skin changed when I detoxed from chemicals and converted to 100% chemical and toxin-free food. Results happen when you feed your cells the nutrients they need. Kick up the dirt, find some food and put it on your face and body! I stopped the Skin War in my body, now it's time to stop the skin war in yours! Step three to Super Power your skin is all about what you feed your skin… and we discuss this next.

Happy detoxing, and may your discoveries be amazing! Every cell in your body will thank you for giving it the fresh and healthy ingredients it needs.

I LOVE YOU, I LOVE YOU, I LOVE YOU! Wow, you gave me my face and my confidence back, thank you! I was prepared for the adjustment period. It never came. I thought my face would act up when I started my period. It didn't. I have not had to go and have a painful injection since I started the Banished™ system. I am going to switch all my body care products from "Big Cosmo" to your wonderful brand. Thanks again,

—Brandi

CHAPTER SIX

Feed: Super Power Your Skin with Real Food

Good health is nothing more than happy cells. Happy cells work at their optimum level to form every healthy organ, system, and dynamic in our bodies. With nutrient-dense products, cells get just what they need for you to feel your best.

We already talked about the havoc chemicals can wreak on your entire system. Now let's focus on healing the body.

So far, we've ditched the chemicals (step one), we are detoxing our systems (step two), let's talk now about step three to Super Power your skin.

Nutrition. Feeding your cells the nutrients they need, in the forms they can use, to function properly. Well-fed skin will protect you. A food-based skin-diet will leave you with a pure radiance and glow. Mother Nature holds in her realms a few dirty secrets of her own. Mother Nature knows beauty and provides real food solutions to prevent aging, acne, congestion, cavities, dandruff, dry/oily skin, and a multitude of other internal and external conditions. Mother Nature's dirty secrets heal, nourish, strengthen and protect with nutrients.

Proper nutrition plays an important role in healing the body because it literally feeds our cells. Cells are basically tiny machines that need the right components to do their job in the same way that your car won't run without gas or will suddenly stop when it doesn't have oil. When they are nourished with food—not chemicals—cells function properly and reproduce new healthy cells. Cells make up tissues. Tissues make up organs. Organs make up systems. Systems make your body function. *Everything* that happens in your body—good or bad—is dependent on the kind of nutrition you give it.

Organically grown food gives our cells the greatest amount of pure nutrients without the chemical impact of conventionally grown foods. And because they are not artificially preserved, organic foods must be eaten more quickly after harvest. Consequently, when you eat organic, you eat fresher food and get greater quantities of the nutrients that deteriorate after harvest.

Vitamin C is a great example of a diminishing nutrient. It oxidizes with time and temperature fluctuations, decreasing the amount we get from citrus fruits, tomatoes, strawberries, etc. Conventionally grown produce is picked well in advance of its natural ripeness so that it can be shipped across the country or the world, which means the countdown to nutritional loss begins long before it arrives on the grocery store shelf. Not only do we get less nutritional bang for our buck, we pay good money to be besieged by the chemical onslaught each bite carries to our cells.

But organic fruits and vegetables and grass-fed or sustainably raised meats give us all their goodness without attacking our endocrine, immune, or any other biological system. In the same way that our bodies are a multi-layered, complex conglomeration of minute interactions among cells, so is every fruit, veggie, or meat a rich, unique combination of vitamins, minerals, antioxidants, proteins, amino acids, sugars, cholesterols, carbohydrates, fats, fiber, and water. Each has its own complexity, which energizes one or more of our biological functions. We need the entire spectrum of nutrition to maintain a healthy body or rebuild a weakened one.

Vitamins are molecules—different ones are necessary for certain biological functions and we need at least thirteen of them—A, C, D, E, K, B1, B2, B3, B6, B12, pantothenic acid, and biotin. We cannot create these in our body, so they must come from our food.

Likewise, there are seven essential minerals—calcium, phosphorus, magnesium, sulfur, sodium, potassium, and chloride. We need minerals like calcium for strong bones, teeth, and nails but also because without it we would have weak muscles and ineffective nerves. We know we need iron for energy and healthy red blood cells. Why? Because red blood cells carry oxygen, which is critical for our survival—not just for breathing, but to create energy by feeding other cellular functions. Each vitamin and mineral plays an important role in the overall scheme of good health.

Most of us know that proteins are contained in meat, but why is protein so important? Because it forms part of our cells and directs growth. Proteins are composed of amino acids, 10 of which are called "essential" and must be acquired daily from food because our bodies can't store them for later use. We eat carbohydrates to burn as a slow-release fuel for energy that supports blood sugar regulation, absorption of calcium, and muscles. Fats—triglycerides, cholesterol, and other essential fatty acids—store energy, act as messengers between cells to assist protein functions, and act as catalysts for growth and immune, reproductive, and metabolic functions. We cannot absorb vitamins A, D, E, and K without fat because these are fat-soluble (stored in fat). And naturally-occurring sugars (monosaccharide) found in fruits, milk, and even grains are critical to having enough energy for our cells to do their jobs.

Omegas:

In recent years, the word "omega" has gained attention and caused a great deal of confusion. We often hear that we should eat more of the good omega-3 foods like fish and fish oils, and walnut, evening primrose, and grapeseed or canola oils. We should also eat omega-6 foods found in nuts and seeds. But what are these omegas?

They are polyunsaturated fats essential for good health, but our body cannot make them so we must get them from food. They help build cells, maintain brain and nerve function, and, increasingly, are thought to protect against heart disease, type 2 diabetes, Alzheimer's disease, and brain function decline.

Antioxidants versus Free Radicals:

Many of us have heard the word a thousand times, but still don't understand it: antioxidants. Often we hear it in connection with free radicals.

Maybe if you're a wild and woolly person, being a free radical might appeal to you. But in your body, just like in society, out of control free radicals create chaos and destruction.

Antioxidants are the micronutrients in many fruits and veggies that give them color. They are also found in seawater plants and seafood. But they have a much more important role as natural chemicals that donate electrons to other atoms and regulate cell damage—preventing it or slowing it down. Naturally occurring antioxidant compounds number in the thousands, but most of us have heard of the most important dietary ones—vitamins A, C, and E, as well as beta-carotene and lycopene.

In the normal course of life, cells are born and die when oxygen interacts with them—a process called oxidation. It is a necessary process that, in balance, results in cell renewal and regeneration, which keeps your body healthy. The way the process stays in balance is through antioxidants, which police the oxidation process. Antioxidants are found in various fruits and vegetables, whole grains and legumes, and nuts. Clearly, antioxidants are vital to health.

Oxidation is normal and happens all day, every day. We never even notice it because our bodies are designed to accommodate it. Each oxidized cell is a free radical, but not every oxidized cell is dangerous because we naturally produce antioxidants (anti = against, oxidant = working with oxygen) that counterbalance it.

Toxins generate free radicals. Remember in Chapter Four where we discussed the extent of pollution that is part and parcel of our everyday lives, in our air, water, and soil? Add cigarette smoke to that list. All of these external influences produce oxidation that results in internal free-radical production.

Free radicals are cells damaged by oxidation. They are missing a molecule so they go crazy looking for a cell to steal that molecule from so they can be whole again. Of course, the cell that loses a molecule is then damaged. Its function is affected and it may even die. If the cells robbed of their molecule by free radicals only died, there wouldn't really be much of a problem. The problem is that these new, altered cells can reproduce quickly in a chain reaction of mutation and malfunction.

The initial stages of cellular-level breakdown are undetectable. Cellular damage is not painful. We never feel cellular mutation or suffocation from a chemical or toxin—it is too minute to notice. By the time we see or feel the damage (aches, pains, rashes, etc.) the damage has affected not just cells, but tissues, organs, and systems. When the tissues are congested and the organs falter, systems begin to show the symptoms of breakdown.

Most of the time, we are past the point of connecting the dots to solve the mystery question: Just how and when did this all begin?

Most likely, the answer is years ago. Years of poor dietary choices, chemical-laden skincare, toxic household cleaners (including laundry detergents), dust, mold, pollution, water contamination, soil pollutants, etc. have caused cellular damage.

Mutated cells have a lifespan. If they reproduce, they spawn a new mutated cell. An overgrowth of mutated cells is how we define cancer. Cancer thrives in a defective, toxic, malnourished environment.

The good news: Our bodies are designed to regenerate. They are forgiving and can heal, but they require the correct nutrients to do so. Organic foods rich in antioxidants control free radical production and reproduction. The top antioxidant performers are cherries, blackberries, blueberries, and cranberries; red, kidney, black, and pinto beans; artichokes, pecans, walnuts, and hazelnuts. Many other foods have wonderful antioxidant properties as well.

Encyclopedias have been written about the functions of all the nutritional components in our foods, but by now you get the picture that though some are critical and others are less essential. Our bodies thrive when we eat a full-spectrum, fresh, and nutrient-dense diet. As resilient as our bodies seem to be, no matter how we abuse them, aim for the best diet you can get—one that is jam-packed with nutrients and tastes good.

What Does Skincare Have to Do with Free Radicals?

When I began my journey creating healthy, real food alternatives to commercial skincare, I knew that the purpose behind each product would be "to improve health." Health is a general term that includes the cells, tissues, organs, and systems of the body. From my nursing background, I know that the individual cells of the body need to be nourished in order for the collective group to function as tissue. The same goes for the tissues. Each individual tissue cell must get the proper nutrition and oxygen in order for the tissues to collectively work properly as an organ.

Obviously, organs work together to function as systems and each individual cell in the system must be nourished. So, what it all comes down to is cellular health. Cells eventually die—some have a lifespan as short as ten hours.

These cells live their intended lifespan (if they are free from disease and defect), regenerate new cells, and then die. The new cells are replicas of the parent cell. If the parent cell is diseased, mutated, or defective, the new cell will also carry this trait. Disease grows from cellular malnutrition, starvation, and suffocation. I have said this before, but it is worth repeating—cancer is just an overgrowth of mutated cells.

The brain is the main component of your nervous system. Brain cells are highly specialized. But did you know that brain cells do not regenerate, that they are with you for your lifetime? Neurons are nerve cells in the brain that are created during fetal development. A few are added during infancy, but new cells are added only to the hippocampus region of the brain during your lifetime.

This is extremely important because as we discussed earlier, chemicals and toxins are lipophilic and can cross the blood-brain barrier. Brain tissue is a fatty tissue; just the type chemicals and toxins love to migrate to for storage. Chemicals and toxins from skincare and diet can cause cell mutation and cell death. Alterations in cells can cause neurological problems—confusion, sluggishness, and a host of other physical symptoms.

Other cells in the body have a lifespan and will regenerate. Below is the average lifespan of the cells of the body:

Red blood cells: 120 days	Lymphocytes: over one year
Other white blood cells: 10 hours	Platelets: 10 days
Brain: lifetime	Bone: 120 days
Colon: 25–35 years	Skin: 19–34 days
Spermatozoa: 2–3 days	Stomach: 2 days

The day I examined my moisturizer bottle and discovered what I had been feeding my cells, I was horrified. How can a cell fed preservatives, chemicals, toxins, and the like, survive? How can it spawn healthy cells? At what point does a nutritionally deprived cell mutate and stop functioning? Can this process be stopped? Can I grow new, healthy cells just by providing the real nutrition the cells need? What about improving my blood supply to increase oxygen supply and utilization? After all, a cell suffocating from a lack of oxygen cannot survive for long.

My next thought was *what does healthy really look like?* I was suffering from acne. My skin was an oil slick. I was getting rashes on my legs and the beginnings of psoriasis had appeared. Is *this* what unhealthy cells look like at the splanchnic (organ) level? My skin is an organ—a very large organ—the largest organ I have. If my skin looks this bad—*WHAT DO MY INTERNAL ORGANS LOOK LIKE???*

Okay, if my skin is congested and functioning abnormally, let's assume my other systems are not functioning well either. Was there any evidence of this in my body? Yes! I was very susceptible to cold and flu viruses. In fact, I was so susceptible that I would recover from one cold and immediately get sick again. Oddly enough, it was at this time that I think I was one of the first to develop the strange symptoms of "bird flu"—sudden onset of severe flu symptoms. It was incredibly horrible.

MY IMMUNE SYSTEM WAS FAILING ME! I no longer had a functioning immune system. Every cell of every organ that made up my immune system was diseased. It wasn't going to change unless I changed my skin's diet. I started making my own carrot-seed moisturizer to give my body a fighting chance at good health.

So, how does my skin look today? I have been making my own skincare products for seven years. It has been at least four years since I bought *any* commercial products. Today, I make everything myself. If I cannot make it, I don't use it. That has been my motivation to figure out how to make each product from food sources. This strict policy is evident in my consistently good health.

Since I changed my skin diet, my acne is gone. I am neither oily nor dry, and my rashes and weird leg irritations are a thing of the past. My complexion glows. I am 46 (while writing this book) and most people guess that I'm still in my early 30s.

Further, my organs and systems must be getting the nutrition they need, because my immune system is back—I no longer get sick as frequently and severely as I used to. I may get the occasional cold, but it is less severe and only lasts two to three days. I conclude that my tissues, organs, and systems are thriving because my cells are receiving the nutrition they need and my blood supply has improved.

Step Three: Super Power Your Skin with Real Food. Mother Nature's Dirty Secrets

Food sources provide the vitamins (A, B, C, D, E, F), minerals (calcium and potassium), essential fatty acids (omega-3, -6, and -9), antioxidants, lipids, oleic acid, linoleic acid, retinoic acid (a metabolite of vitamin A), phytosterols, and capsicum. FOOD. HEALS. CELLS.

Not only do food sources provide nutrition, they protect against bacteria, viruses, and fungus. Food regenerates skin cells more rapidly, reduces scarring, and promotes healing. It can reduce the sensation of pain and inflammation and improve blood supply by bolstering the functioning of the red blood cells. Food sources hydrate the cells, which increases cellular activity. Many essential oils are also cytophylactic, meaning they promote the regeneration of healthy cells and keep existing cells and tissues vibrant.

Remember when we talked about the importance of water in Chapter Five? Food sources hydrate the cells, which increases cellular activity.

You will find that your largest organ—your mighty skin—will thrive on a food-based diet. Once freed from preservatives, chemicals, and toxins, your cells will be nourished, hydrated, oxygenated, and produce healthier cells. They will live their intended lifespan and function optimally. Mutated cells do not thrive in an environment where healthy cells reign.

I am not suggesting cancer will "go away" by changing your skincare. I am suggesting that cells starting to mutate may not progress any further; that healthy cells will replace mutated cells by the law of survival of the fittest, and if your cells are healthy, the chance for mutations to grow will be lessened.

I have researched thousands of natural alternatives—oils, essential oils, herbs, tinctures, infusions, clays, flowers, plants, and foods. From this extensive research, I discovered that the healing properties of all of these sources work both inside and outside of the body.

I love formulating and tailoring ingredients to target certain problems. It's an art. It's a science. It's a little voodoo. It's a little luck. It took a lot of faith—so much faith that before I research ingredients for *any* product, I always ask for guidance from the Hand Above.

What I learned along the way is that natural sources rooted in the earth provide profound healing powers and properties that our bodies literally soak up, not just to survive, but to thrive. Knowing the healing properties of these God-given sources is important. Why does Big Cosmo not want you to feed your skin food? Because real food costs a lot more money than water and chemicals. Big Cosmo is about mass producing large quantities of cheap products to make the biggest buck. To mass produce, they must use chemical preservatives to prolong the shelf life. It is a vicious cycle with no concern for your long-term health.

Super Power Foods for Your Skin

OILS, ESSENTIAL OILS, FOODS, AND HERBS

Baobab Oil is very rich in vitamins A, D, E, and F; oleic acid; linoleic acid; and omega-3, -6 and -9 fatty acids. Baobab oil has been used for centuries to improve skin elasticity and encourage skin cell regeneration. It is easily and quickly absorbed and does not clog pores. The omega fats in the oil make it useful in treating acne, eczema, and psoriasis. It is also known to reduce scarring from acne, heal existing scars and stretch marks, reduce signs of aging, and improve skin tone.

Beeswax (pure, unfiltered) provides excellent, breathable protection against the natural elements. It has healing and antiseptic properties and will not clog pores.

Bergamot essential oil's antibacterial and drying properties make it an ideal spot treatment for existing blemishes, while its antiseptic quality and ability to promote skin growth make it perfect for treating acne.

Borage seed oil has the highest concentration of naturally occurring gamma-linolenic acid (GLA), higher than any other plant source! Borage seed oil has been used with positive results for many different skin disorders including psoriasis, eczema, acne, rosacea, and prematurely matured skin.

Calendula oil contains a high level of carotenoids in its chemical composition and has excellent re-epithelizing (covering with new epithelial tissue) properties, making it ideal for general healing as well as healing wounds. Its superior antimicrobial and antioxidizing properties help prevent infection and promote healing.

Carrot seed essential oil regenerates the epidermal skin cells and stimulates cell growth. It effectively rejuvenates aged, tired, dehydrated, and damaged skin. Carrot seeds are rich in beta-carotene as well as vitamins B, C, D, and E, and improve the function of red blood cells, thereby improving the tone and elasticity of the skin.

Cayenne pepper is high in vitamins A, C, and B complex, calcium, and potassium. Cayenne pepper has many amazing properties including pain and inflammation relief. Applying cayenne pepper topically can be amazing for your skin—it improves both minor and major blemishes as well as improves your skin's look and feel. Applied topically, cayenne pepper increases blood flow to the skin, which increases the delivery of oxygen and many essential nutrients that aid in healing. Capsicum—the ingredient in cayenne peppers that makes them hot—has mild antibacterial properties and may help kill some of the bacteria that cause acne.

Chamomile essential oil disinfects and has vulnerary (wound healing), cicatrisant (scar healing), and antiseptic properties that promote skin healing and prevent scar tissue formation.

Citronella essential oil has analgesic, antibacterial, antifungal, antiseptic, astringent, and tonic properties that make it extremely effective against acne.

Clove bud essential oil has potent purifying, analgesic, and anti-inflammatory properties. It is very strong and acts very quickly. It can be used to relieve painful acne sores and reduce redness and swelling.

Cypress essential oil contains antiseptic and antibacterial properties to help prevent infections and promote skin healing.

Emu oil contains a complete balance of essential fatty acids (omega-3, -6, and -9), which plays a part in the regeneration of healthy new skin cells. Natural lipids found in emu oil match that of human skin, and replenishing these lipids helps replenish skin from the inside out. Emu oil supports our skin's natural stimulation of proteins, resulting in faster rejuvenation.

Evening primrose oil is a rich source of GLA—an omega-6 fatty acid—that effectively treats acne, rosacea, signs of aging, and eczema.

Frankincense essential oil has incredible properties for skin rejuvenation and it helps to prevent or fade scars. It is cytophylactic and promotes the production of leucocytes (white blood cells). One of its most valuable and interesting properties is as a cicatrisant—it helps fade scars left by boils, acne, or pox.

Geranium essential oil is often used to soothe inflamed and irritated skin due to its healing and analgesic properties. It increases blood circulation and skin elasticity. When added to massage oil, geranium oil reduces dryness and sagging by encouraging moisture retention in the skin. When added as an ingredient to skin moisturizers and toners, this botanical also helps fight wrinkles.

Helichrysum essential oil contains anti-inflammatory and tissue-regenerating properties. It soothes irritated skin and promotes healing of damaged tissues.

Hemp seed oil is anti-inflammatory agent with anti-aging properties. It balances dry skin, helps heal skin lesions, contains antioxidants, and balances moisture. This oil is non-greasy and readily absorbs into the pores. It is an emollient—a moisturizer that also has rejuvenating properties for the skin.

Jojoba oil's unique chemical makeup mimics the sebum naturally present on human skin. Jojoba is odorless, non-greasy, a carrier of vitamin E, and an antioxidant. It is an extremely efficient noncomedogenic (preventing formation of blackheads) moisture regulator—it penetrates the skin without blocking the pores. Because it also reduces sebum production and protects the skin from bacteria, jojoba oil can also effectively treat acne.

Lavender essential oil is highly effective via a number of healing properties. It soothes pain, prevents bacterial infection, aids in scar-free healing and has soothing, calming, and restorative properties. It can even replace scars with a new layer of skin.

Menthol crystals applied topically to an area affected by acne will activate cold-sensitive receptors in skin, causing a cooling sensation that overrides the irritation from swollen and inflamed blemishes. Because of this property, they effectively reduce pain and tenderness.

Myrrh essential oil's soothing and astringent qualities make it excellent for relieving a wide variety of skin conditions including acne outbreaks, sensitive, oily, or dry skin; and wrinkled, chapped, or cracked skin. Myrrh helps scars and age spots fade, and is excellent for treating skin conditions like eczema and rashes. Myrrh is also a skin tonic—it strengthens and enlivens skin cells.

Neroli essential oil is an effective essential treatment for scars and rejuvenating mature skin.

Pomegranate seed oil deeply nourishes the outer epidermal layer and provides powerful antioxidants. Pomegranate seed oil's antioxidants neutralize free radicals that otherwise cause skin damage and visible signs of aging. Cold-pressed organic seeds of the pomegranate fruit are naturally high in flavonoids as well as punicic and ellagic acids. Because of these key properties, pomegranate seed oil is used to heal, protect, and moisturize dry, cracked, mature, and irritated skin. It also restores skin elasticity and is beneficial for eczema, psoriasis, and other skin ailments.

Pumpkin seed oil is especially effective in combating fine lines, superficial dryness, and moisture loss. Pumpkin seed oil is nourishing for aging skin because of its high levels of fatty acids, protein, zinc, and polyunsaturated fats.

Red thyme essential oil has antiseptic, disinfectant, analgesic, antibacterial, antifungal, anti-inflammatory, and antimicrobial properties superior for skin healing.

Rosehip seed oil (Rosa Mosqueta or *Rosa rubiginosa)* is the only vegetable oil that contains natural retinoic acid. It is the best vegetable source of omega-3 as well as a great source of omega-6. Recent studies have shown that rosehip seed oil regenerates the skin and reduces scars. Some studies have shown that it can reduce the appearance of sunspots, promote skin elasticity, smooth wrinkles, and improve skin tone and quality.

Sea buckthorn oil is highly prized oil typically used to treat damaged skin, ulcerations, scar tissue, wrinkles and eczema. The high content of fat-soluble vitamins (A, E) and nutrients (EFAs, phytosterols) makes sea buckthorn an indispensable ingredient for restorative, anti-aging, and revitalizing skin care. Sea buckthorn oil is superior for nourishing, revitalizing, and restoring aging skin.

Tamanu oil has been shown to heal damaged and scarred skin. The ability of tamanu oil to heal the skin surpasses that of most (if not all) modern-day skin care products. Scientific studies show that tamanu oil is a significant healing agent because of its ability to produce new skin tissue and because of its anti-inflammatory, anti-neuralgic (pain reducing), antibiotic, and antioxidant properties for younger skin.

CLAYS

Bentonite clay contains over 70 trace minerals. It is one of the most powerful and effective healing clays for superficial maladies. Bentonite clay contains the minerals your teeth need to re-mineralize and strengthen them. Over time, your teeth lose minerals in the latticework of the enamel. Demineralized teeth are sensitive and if demineralization continues, cavities result. I created Dirty Mouth Toothpowder with bentonite clay to help remineralize teeth back to health! Mother Nature Knows Best, and gives us earthly solutions for real health issues.

Diatomaceous earth clay comes from diatoms—microscopic one-celled algae that are abundant in oceans and lakes. When oceans and lake beds dry up over eons, the fossilized shells of the diatoms remain. Therefore, diatomaceous earth is marine-based. The remaining sediment is harvested and milled into a fine powder. This clay is highly absorbent and is an opacifying agent that makes solutions less transparent. In skin-food cosmetic terms that means it lightens the appearance of blemishes.

French green clay is incredibly absorbent and brings fresh blood to damaged skin cells, revitalizing complexions and tightening pores. Its anti-inflammatory and cleansing properties help reduce acne.

Fuller's earth clay is also very absorbent clay that draws oil out of the skin, making it perfect for those with oily skin or who are prone to acne.

Kaolin clays (yellow, pink, white, and red) are very gentle and absorbent clays. Kaolin clays gently draw impurities from the skin without removing the natural oils. They reduce sebum production, the main contributor to greasy skin. They help soothe and heal, as well as purify and nourish all skin types. They also serve as an exfoliant and cleanser, and enhance blood circulation.

I do not believe in using preservatives. Fresh is best and I always give my skin the healthiest ingredients possible. When my skin soaks up the nutrients from these ingredients, I can feel and see a difference.

My fine lines have faded because my cells are no longer dehydrated. My complexion glows because my cells are no longer starving for oxygen—they live in a well-oxygenated environment with a vast blood supply. My skin feels full and plump because my cells are fed well and thoroughly nourished. My skin conditions have gone away because my cells are not congested and can get rid of their waste products. Free radicals are neutralized quickly by the numerous antioxidants in my bloodstream.

I continue to look and feel younger because my cells are regenerating faster and producing healthy young cells. My cells are living a full life and my tissues, organs, and systems are proof that what you put on your skin does matter. I have Super Powered my skin with real food. Because Mother Nature Knows Beauty!

For your cells to be their best, look first at the rudimentary medicine chest right at your fingertips.

Skin Remedies You Can Find in Your Kitchen: Where Do YOU Start?

Home is where the heart is and where health begins. I started my skincare reform in my kitchen—and you can too!

The following foods are basic but will get the job done until you are ready to add more nutrients and improve your results.

Extra virgin olive oil, coconut oil, macadamia nut oil, and almond oil are all wonderful, nutrient-dense oils that can be found in most grocery stores. They make wonderful cleansers, makeup removers, and moisturizers.

Baking soda under the arms does a great job at reducing wetness from sweating in a hot kitchen—dab a little under there instead of toxic deodorant or antiperspirant. Coconut oil does a great job at minimizing odor—add a little under the arms while you whip up your favorite treat. Or invest in StickUp 100% natural deodorant to make your life a little easier!

Baking soda has been used for years in place of toothpaste. Apple cider vinegar is an excellent facial toner. Honey, avocado, and eggs are excellent facial masks. Sugar is a great exfoliator.

While organic oils, baking soda, sugar, and apple cider vinegar are great places to start, eventually you may want more—more anti-aging, nutrition, healing, detox, toning, vitamins, omegas, and antioxidants. Or you may want less—fewer wrinkles, discolorations, acne, less scarring, bacteria, inflammation, and congestion. And you probably will want everything faster—faster healing, improvement, and results.

I have created more than 100 chemical-free alternatives to commercial skincare, hair products, dental care, and makeup. Because I have fully researched each and every ingredient I use, I am able to create products that heal the cells of the body so the body can repair itself and improve functionality. I make it easy to stay beautiful and healthy without harming your body.

☞☞☞

This book is about healing the body with the proper nutrients. I have provided a lot of information about the skin and the importance of the skin-food that goes on it.

Equally important, the food you put into your body must provide real nutrients. Healing the gut is a great place to start. Poor nutrition cripples your gut's ability to work easily, efficiently, and fully. A poorly functioning gut leads to inflammatory processes that affect every organ of the body. Modern medicine has acknowledged that inflammation is the root cause of nearly every disease.

If you are truly interested in healing the body from the inside as well as the outside, I highly recommend and urge you to read *Purely Primal Skincare* by Liz Wolfe. I am honored to have contributed to the book as the guest expert, offering insight about natural skincare solutions.

Liz has a wealth of knowledge and shares it in numerous ways: as a nutrition coach and podcaster, a magazine columnist, a Nutritional Therapy Practitioner (NTP™) certified by the Nutritional Therapy Association, a public health student, and an advocate.

In *Purely Primal Skincare*, Liz offers solutions for better health and living:

> ❯ Why **almost everyone needs digestive help**, and how to get it

> ❯ The nutrients you need for beautiful skin, lovely hair, and a radiant body, and where to find them

> ❯ Unexpected **superfoods** that are critical for skin wellness ("conventional wisdom" not welcome!)

> ❯ How to **get nutrients where they need to go**

> ❯ How to ditch toxins in food, your body, and your body care routine!

> ❯ The **best products on the planet** for cleansing and nourishing the skin (hint: there are NO unpronounceable ingredients or unnecessary chemicals!)

> ❯ Alternatives to conventional makeup, hair dyes, and hair care products

> ❯ Strategies for improving cellulite

> ❯ Tips for smart intimate and feminine care

Find *Purely Primal Skincare* at http://bit.ly/WCXWdJ.

Healthy Skin Is Radiant and Glowing
Give Your Skin Super Powers

That skin can be your skin! Even persistent, common conditions that many adults suffer with can be resolved with nutrient-dense skincare. Many people have completely eliminated itching, breakouts, and scarring by using our pure ingredients that are free of toxins. Mother Nature Super Powers your skin. Trust Mother Nature, she has your health in mind. She will provide you with skin that is radiant and glowing!

It's not too often I've come across a skincare product that is not only suitable for my skin, but also meets my criteria of being organic, all-natural, and free of harsh chemicals. I have had chronic, cystic acne and excessively oily skin since I was 9 years old (I'm 31 now). I had seen dermatologists for years and tried every acne prescription available. I was tired of wasting money and becoming more and more disheartened every time I looked in the mirror. It was both emotionally and physically painful. I purchased your Carrot Seed Cleanser about a month and a half ago. I LOVE it! My skin is clear—seriously! Thanks so much for creating such a great product that works not just for my skin, but the Primal lifestyle as a whole.

——Shannon

CHAPTER SEVEN

Heal: Super Power Your Recovery from Acne, Rosacea, Psoriasis and Perioral Dermatitis

Are you suffering from toxic overload from your skincare? Your skincare products could be causing or contributing to your acne, sneezing, watery eyes, oily skin, dry skin, rashes, irritation, blotchiness, redness, swelling, rosacea, eczema, psoriasis, dermatitis, or dull, saggy and lifeless skin.

ere we are, at the point of addressing a few common but very distressing skin issues. Most of us know someone who suffers from perioral dermatitis, psoriasis, rosacea, or adult acne—many of us suffer from these ourselves. You'll remember my own story of suffering acne for years before discovering that *adding* oil to my skin helped it stop going into overdrive oil production because it was constantly robbed of its natural oil by the commercial (and very expensive) skincare products I was using.

Unfortunately, many of the chemicals used in Big Cosmo products are harsh skin and internal irritants. Any inflammatory response causes a trifecta of reactions in your body. As mentioned earlier, almost all health conditions are inflammatory in nature— it is very possible that skin conditions could also be linked to an inflammatory response as well. Irritants cause numerous reactions invisible to the naked eye. What we may see on the outside as a result of the inflammatory response is acne, rosacea, eczema, psoriasis, and more.

Using commercial skincare products with harsh chemicals can be similar to the effects oral medications have on the body. They can produce unwanted "side effects" in our bodies, causing us to then add more arsenal to the fire. For instance, using an anti-aging cream to prevent wrinkles may contain ingredients that disrupt the function of your cells, causing inflammation and cellular changes. What you may witness is acne or breakouts—now you must add another topical (or medication) to treat the breakouts. That topical causes dry, irritated skin. Back to the cosmetic counter you go. Welcome to the Big Cosmo Pharm—you now need more bottles of chemical irritants to treat the "side effects" of their miracle cure. If you suffer from any skin condition, take a closer look at your Big Cosmo bottles and read the ingredients. Harsh chemicals might be the source of evil causing, or contributing to your skin condition.

This chapter will help you learn how to Super Power your recovery from skin conditions, help prevent them or at least head them off at the pass while the conditions are still new and easily changed.

According to the government's website for women's health,[10] normal cosmetics can contain any one the 5,000 fragrances or

---

10 http://www.womenshealth.gov/publications/our-publications/

preservatives allowed by law—in fact, they are the *main ingredients* in cosmetics. Fragrances are often made up of chemicals that irritate the skin and lungs, and many components in fragrance promote acne breakouts. Worse than just being exposed to these toxins, consider the little-known fact that the US Food and Drug Administration (FDA) do not require manufacturers to list them by name on the label. If you are sensitive or allergic to a fragrance, you will never be able to find out exactly which ingredient causes you difficulty, or even avoid it once you know it's a problem.

Preservatives control the growth of fungus and bacteria and prevent damage from exposure to light or air. But preservatives are one of the worst culprits for skin irritation or infection.

Phthalates are added as a softener for many commercial cosmetics. In addition to giving your favorite lotion a creamy feel, phthalates are also irritants that can cause asthma and allergies, especially in children.

Even prenatal exposure to some chemicals will predispose children to skin irritations. A 2007 study[11] found that the risk of children developing eczema by two years old increased by 52 percent when pregnant mothers used products containing butyl benzyl phthalate (BBzP), a common chemical in soap and shampoo.

Do I need to repeat one more time that using commercial skin-care products will promote the causes of acne, rosacea, psoriasis or perioral dermatitis? You may be sick of hearing me say it, but the message is still so critical to understand—your *healthy* body would not feel the need to create these compensatory, defensive conditions. Super Power skin is fed nutrients from Mother Nature. Increased clean blood flow carries oxygen rich blood cells to the tissues. The cells can rid themselves of waste products, nutrients can

---

11 http://www.pediatricsdigest.mobi/content/121/2/e260.short

penetrate the surface, cells live their intended lifespan and reproduce healthy cells. These four conditions are just a few of the many
ways your skin will tell you that something is definitely not cool in
your interior landscape.

ADULT ACNE

What it is: Just like juvenile acne, the sebaceous glands over-
produce the sebum that clogs skin pores. These congested pores
attract bacteria, which leads to inflammation. Acne is the most
common skin condition for both teens and adults, but most don't
know what the causes it. Many people with acne have unsuccess-
fully tried over-the-counter products as well as laser therapy, drug
therapy (including Accutane), antibiotics, hormone therapy, and
corticosteroids.

Why it is: An underlying hormonal imbalance causes overproduction of male hormones called androgens, but out of balance
estrogen can also be the initiating culprit. Hormonal blood levels
are one source, but steroidal medications and commercial cosmetics
also promote the hormone imbalance that causes acne. Pregnancy,
perimenopause, and menopause are prime times for women to have
breakouts.

Poor digestion plays a very big role in the overproduction of
sebum as well as poor lymph flow, which promotes weak toxin
removal. Along with the toxic ingredients in commercial skincare,
a leaky gut, inflammatory foods, hormonal imbalances, food sensitivities, and nutritional deficiencies can all cause acne. *Purely Primal
Skincare* is a great resource for healing your gut, and using pure
skincare products will eliminate the daily doses of toxins that lead

to skin reactions. Using natural skincare products gives your pores time to breathe and your skin cells time to heal.

Let's go back to my story as an example. I suffered from acne from the time I was a teen until I was forty years old. I can tell you, I tried everything on the market including medical interventions, over-the-counter topical medications, and home remedies. In the twenty-seven years I suffered from acne, not once did any physician talk to me about my diet.

There are certain foods that can cause acne and if eliminated, the acne may resolve. After all, according to The Center for Food Allergies, "A majority of acne cases, as well as many other skin blemishes, are caused by food allergies. Hormone imbalances may also play a role, but are largely overrated."[12]

These are the worst culprits:

> **Dairy**—Very high possibility

> **Nightshades**—Potatoes, tomatoes, sweet and hot peppers, eggplant, tomatillos, tamarios, pepinos, pimentos, paprika, and cayenne peppers

> **Nuts**

> **Gluten**

> **Sugar**—Due to a spike in insulin

Did you know that the benzoyl peroxide widely used in acne products is a *toxic* ingredient that may promote tumor formation and DNA mutations or damage? The Material Safety Data Sheet (MSDS) says it can cause irritation in the eyes or skin, and respiratory and/or digestive tracts.[13]

---

12 http://www.centerforfoodallergies.com/acne.htm
13 https://www.nwmissouri.edu/naturalsciences/sds/b/Benzoyl%20peroxide.pdf

If you are pregnant, avoiding benzoyl peroxide is a must. If you care about animal cruelty, you have another reason to avoid products with this ingredient because researchers use animals to test it.

What to do: Simplify and purify. Go out into the sun and let its rays promote vitamin D production in your body. Vitamin D is a natural antibiotic, perfect for fighting the bacteria in those clogged pores. It plays a huge role in the healthy function of all your organs, and you know by now that organ malfunction—in this case, skin afflicted with acne—is a result of cellular damage. Walking out your front door and soaking up some rays is the simplest treatment for acne. And you might even sweat a little, pushing out a few more toxins that way.

As much as possible, eliminate toxins from your environment. But please also remember that foods can cause or worsen *all* of the above conditions. Acne, psoriasis, etc. may be your skin's reaction to the chemicals you smear on it every day, or it may be a sign that your gut lacks the healthy bacterial flora necessary for good digestion and absorption of nutrients.

Many foods are inflammatory and provoke skin reactions. Consider an elimination diet to see if symptoms improve or resolve. A wonderful resource for understanding the elimination diet is http://www.dermaharmony.com/skinnutrition/eliminationdiet-forskinconditions.aspx.

Using an elimination diet, remove inflammatory foods like these:

> **Food additives**—Includes monosodium glutamate (MSG), artificial sweeteners, preservatives, artificial flavors, and artificial colorings

> **Alcohol**—Beer, wine, and spirits (hard alcohol), vanilla extract, Angostura bitters, mouthwash, cough medicine, and some homeopathic remedies

> **Citrus fruits**—Oranges, tangerines, grapefruit, limes, lemons, kumquats, and others

> **Shellfish**—Lobster, crab, mussels, clams, scallops, etc.

> **Nuts**—Cashews, pecans, walnuts, pistachios, and other tree nuts, plus groundnuts like peanuts

> **Corn**—Corn oil, high-fructose corn syrup, vegetable oil, corn chips, popcorn, cornstarch, and the multitude of products that contain this common inflammatory food. For a surprising list, check out this website: http://www.cornallergens.com/list/corn-allergen-list.php.

> **Dairy**—Milk, cream, butter, cheese, cottage cheese, whey, yogurt, kefir, sour cream, ice cream, and dulce de leche

> **Eggs**—Both yolk and whites

> **Gluten**—A protein found in grains of the wheat tribe (wheat, Kamut, spelt, triticale, barley, rye, and some oats), but also present in other foods because of contamination with these grains. Pasta, flour, bread, cereal, and crackers all contain gluten.

> **Soy**—Soybeans, tofu, tempeh, edamame, soy sauce, tamari, soy milk, and textured soy protein

> **Sweeteners**—Honey, maple syrup, sugars (white and brown), fructose, dextrose, and maltose

Our bodies are a complex and gorgeous interplay of innumerable factors. It is impossible to separate one from the rest, but by eliminating one thing at a time, we can control and improve what we give our bodies to work with to heal and be strong.

I created the Banished and Beyond Face Primal Package just for acne-prone skin. Made from real food sources, oils, and essential oils, it will encourage the skin to function normally and not strip the skin of its natural, protective oils. One of my most popular products is the Banished Blemish Serum, made with an infusion of cayenne pepper. This is a spot treatment for blemishes that reduces their lifespan. Cayenne pepper is one of Mother Nature's best-kept secrets and I discovered that adding it to the serum increases the blood flow to the breakout, helping it heal more quickly. The added essential oils target inflammation, redness, and scarring. These oils also improve healing. I have had numerous breakouts heal overnight with just one application. It's amazing how well-fed skin heals much faster than skin that is starving for nutrients.

ROSACEA

What it is: A recurring or chronic redness, usually on the face (even in the eyes), it can affect other areas of the upper body like the scalp, ears, neck, and chest. Symptoms vary from simple redness to inflammation to eruptions that range from spots to actual pustules that can sting or itch. Though rosacea usually breaks out then goes away, each occurrence is worse than the prior one. Left untreated, it can change the texture of the skin, making it thick and bumpy, or create swelling that requires surgery.

Why it is: Rosacea is an inflammatory condition that worsens over time. Extremes seem to trigger it, whether they are heavy stress, extreme temperatures, very spicy foods, or intense emotions.

What to do: Eliminate toxins and irritants from your skincare by moisturizing with coconut oil. This simple and pure oil will provide more healing than any commercial moisturizer containing water, alcohol, fragrance, and other endocrine disruptors that irritate the skin and strip away natural oils while they interrupt normal hormone production and function.

You should also heal your gut and digestive tract so you release the toxins stored there, and increase your absorption of nutrients from food. It goes without saying that a healthy diet, free of chemicals and foods to which you might be sensitive, is fundamental to reducing the inflammation caused by rosacea. *Purely Primal Skincare* I mentioned earlier also has a lot of great information on this subject.

From my line of products, I highly recommend the Infiniti Primal Face Package—it's loaded with oils and essential oils that help heal rosacea and help reduce inflammation and redness. It will also help diminish scarring and reduce signs of aging (help fade fine lines, wrinkles, and discolorations).

PSORIASIS

What it is: Psoriasis is a perfect example of an afflicted and weakened immune system. The main symptoms are chronic or intermittent inflammation that leads to scaling (flaking) skin, usually around pressure points on the body (knuckles, knees, and elbows). But it can also affect the scalp, arms and legs, the trunk, nails on both hands and feet, and the external sex organs.

Skin cells begin to grow rampantly, and in a few days as many cells form as would normally form in a few weeks. But because there's no time for your body to get rid of the extra cells, they build up on your skin's surface, forming lesions.

In addition to lesions, psoriasis can cause candida—a fungal/yeast infection that develops when a weakened immune system allows the yeast to get out of control.

Why it is: Digestive problems, inflammation, and a sensitive or hyperactive immune response are common initiators of psoriasis outbreaks. Stress is usually a factor, but outbreaks may also be caused by food and gluten allergies. A mineral deficiency—usually zinc—can trigger an outbreak and may include a concomitant drop in gastric hydrochloric acid.

What to do: Because psoriasis is stress-based, you have to reduce stress to control recurrences. Whether you do it through meditation, walks, or music, learning how to calm yourself internally will go miles in any kind of healing, but with psoriasis it is so important. Taking a walk outside in the sunlight helps reduce stress and gives your skin the vitamin D it needs to heal. According to Anthony Norman, a dedicated researcher and expert on vitamin D[14], this vitamin affects many of our organs, and our skin is the largest of them.

Epsom salt baths or bathing in salt water also helps because it reduces inflammation, removes scales, and eases itching.

I cannot state enough how important it is to eat a nutrient-dense

---

14 http://phys.org/news142791717.html#jCp

diet. You need superfoods, in their purest form, to provide the necessary components that will strengthen your immune system again and give balanced doses of natural minerals like zinc.

Finally, it would also be beneficial to use toxin-free skincare products—especially those that contain no fragrances or perfumes—to avoid the allergens commercial products contain. Soaps, moisturizers, shampoo, conditioners, shaving creams, makeup, deodorant, and styling products all contain ingredients that can irritate or exaggerate psoriasis.

I make all of my products from ingredients that heal the body; therefore, all Primal Life Organics Skin-Food can help improve outbreaks of psoriasis.

PERIORAL DERMATITIS

What it is: Perioral dermatitis (PD) is a fairly common facial skin problem in which itchy, small red bumps form around the mouth and spread to the chin, upper lip, and cheeks. The tissue that borders the lips is typically not affected, although it may be pink, dry, and flaky.

Periocular dermatitis is the same disorder but affects the areas around the nose, eyelids, genitals, and anus.

PD primarily affects women and is considered a variant of rosacea. Those susceptible to PD often suffer from oily skin in the affected area.

Why it is: As with the other issues I have discussed, PD has many possible causes. Diet and certain trigger foods are a possibility. Because of their chemical components, commercial cosmetics and skincare products—especially face creams, makeup, sunscreen, and face washes—can also be a cause. Products containing petrolatum, paraffin, or isopropyl myristate are common triggers for PD, as are topical steroids. Interestingly, fluorinated toothpaste and oral contraceptives are also common causes of PD.

What to do: The best treatment is always to eliminate the trigger—most likely, products that you apply to your skin.

Pure, 100 percent natural ingredients tend to be very gentle and work with the body, not against it. Replacing the chemicals with real food sources allows the cells to heal and function properly. Ingredients that improve healing, diminish scarring, provide vitamins, antioxidants, and omegas, and increase cellular regeneration will improve PD fairly rapidly.

Most times, we are led to believe there is nothing we can do about a condition. The truth of the matter is this: If I feed my body the food it needs for cellular survival, my body will function normally and my skin will be radiant and glowing.

I have had numerous reports of women who have suffered years with PD and have had no relief. I typically recommend the Primal Life Organics Infiniti Face Moisturizer or our Beyond Face Moisturizer because both of these products contain the vitamins, essential fatty acids, and antioxidants as well as anti-inflammatory, antimicrobial, antioxidizing, and cell regenerating properties to which PD responds so well.

$$\backsim \backsim \backsim$$

We change our diets to improve how we absorb and use nutrients on the inside, and we change our skincare products to feed and strengthen our bodies from the outside. Pregnancy offers women the opportunity to nurture and nourish two bodies at one time, and set their children up for a lifetime of greater freedom from health concerns. Yes, you can (and will) Super Power your uterus too!

_____

I am 41 and have struggled with adult acne since age 25. I've tried almost all the high end makeup companies' acne programs and skincare regimes, and have used over-the-counter products and prescription medications, including Accutane, to keep it at bay. I tried OCM, neem oil, and tea tree. A few months ago the cystic acne came back with a vengeance. Being new to Paleo and trying to be more conscious about what my family of 10 puts on our skin, I decided to give the Banished and Beyond Package a try. It has well exceeded my expectations! There was no detox period for me, thankfully, and I never had the red, itchy, peeling, burning skin that I experienced with almost everything else. My old scars are fading faster than I thought possible and this has totally regulated my over-active oily t-zone/dry cheeks issues. The smell is fantastic and I can't imagine ever going back to the harsh chemical laden products. Thank you so much for creating these products. I've been telling friends and family, too!

—Jennifer K.

CHAPTER EIGHT

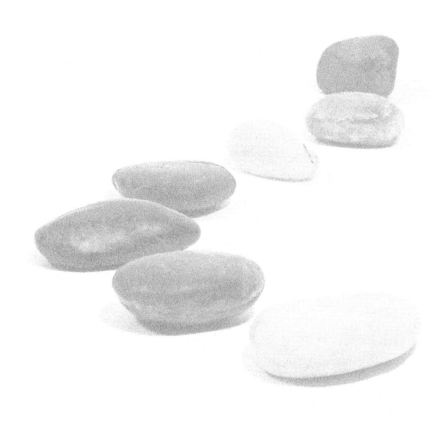

Protect: Super Power Your Uterus for a Healthy Pregnancy

"The Environmental Working Group, in partnership with Rachel's Network, commissioned five laboratories in the US, Canada, and Europe to analyze umbilical cord blood collected from 10 minority infants born in 2007 and 2008. Collectively, the labs identified up to 232 industrial compounds and pollutants in these babies, finding complex mixtures of compounds in each infant."[1]

Aren't you amazed to see your skin stretch and stretch to accommodate your developing baby? It's nearly miraculous what women's bodies are capable of—how they change to grow a baby, feed that baby, then revert again to a no-baby state. I'm still in awe, six years after having gone through the process myself for the first time.

---

[1] This research demonstrates that industrial chemicals cross the placenta in large numbers to contaminate a baby even before the moment of birth.

Pregnancy is the first time many of us begin to question the purity of the food we're eating—the food that we're now using to feed our precious developing babies. We often make changes like expanding our household budget to cover the cost of going organic. We begin to pore over those ingredient labels. And we begin to notice that the ingredients in some of those so-called "natural" and "healthy" food and beauty products don't sound healthy at all. Our new awareness has us wondering how the products we have been using will affect our precious cargo.

As you know by now, that's certainly what happened to me—I was shocked to see the long list of known toxins in my moisturizer, and I refused to use it in order to protect my growing baby. Before that moment, even though my husband and I were living a healthy lifestyle, I'd never thought to question the "healthy" label on our skincare products. But my mysterious miscarriage only 10 weeks earlier had made me hypervigilant, compelling me to search for non-chemical skincare products safe to use during pregnancy.

As I began to educate myself, I realized that those lipophilic, lab-formulated chemicals weren't just going to be cycling through my body. Because they are fat-soluble, they can easily cross the placental barrier. My developing baby—a tiny bundle of growing nerve fibers at that point—was being exposed to hundreds, possibly thousands of chemicals, most of them known neurotoxins and cell mutagens.

This thought alone scared the pants right off of me. What I was learning was truly making me fear for my innocent child. And with good reason: As the EWG reports, toxins found in foods and environmental sources have been identified in the placental cord blood of newborn babies. The same is true for the thousands of chemicals added to skincare products.

I had used hundreds of chemical-laden skincare products in my days prior to converting to a Paleo lifestyle. I can tell you for a fact, NOT ONE product carried this warning:

Caution, this product contains chemicals that can cause birth defects, neurological damage, cell mutations, and possible fetal death.

Not one—even though every one of these products contained preservatives, emulsifiers, thickening agents, foaming agents, and numerous other unnecessary evils. Skincare safe enough for pregnancy did not exist.

So I took matters into my own hands, literally.

I created the one all-natural moisturizer I knew would protect my baby while nourishing my belly's stretching skin. To my trained nurse's mind, nothing could be better than nature's own oils and essential oils, and "natural" *should* mean that the product would sustain my skin with 100 percent pronounceable ingredients like coconut, versus unpronounceable and mysterious unknowns like distearyldimonium chloride.

No product made for pregnant women should contain parabens, synthetic fragrances, phthalates, propylene glycol, lead, petrochemicals, sodium laurel sulfate, chemical preservatives, or 1,4 Dioxane. All of these are neurotoxins that affect the fetal neurological system (encompassing its brain, spinal cord, and peripheral nervous system) at a time when it is most vulnerable.

Beyond this list of known toxins, there are a couple of other things to watch out for in selecting your products. Essential oils are powerful, but not all essential oils are created equal. Please check yours to confirm that they do not contain additives or preservatives, linalool, pesticides, or herbicide residues, and look for high quality therapeutic-grade essential oils like those we use at Primal Life Organics—these will be distilled at low temperatures and low pressure from plant material to prevent distorting their chemical balance and composition.

Although they are natural, some natural oils/essential oils are not suitable for use while growing a baby. Here are a few to avoid, and why:

OIL	EFFECT
Angelica	Emmenagogue (induces menstruation)
Anise seed oil	Has hormone-like effect
Basil	Emmenagogue
Calamus	Neurotoxin (hurts the nervous system)
Camphor	Neurotoxin
Carrot seed; carotene	Possible link to birth defects; possible emmenagogue
Cedarwood	Emmenagogue
Clary sage	Emmenagogue
Fennel oil	Has hormone-like effect; neurotoxin
Ginger	Emmenagogue
Hyssop	Neurotoxin
Jasmine	Emmenagogue
Juniper berry	Emmenagogue
Mugwort	Abortifacient (induces abortions)
Myrrh	Emmenagogue

OIL	EFFECT
Parsley seed	Abortifacient
Pennyroyal	Abortifacient
Rue	Abortifacient
Sage	Neurotoxin, abortifacient, emmenagogue
Sassafras	Abortifacient
Savin	Emmenagogue
Sweet marjoram	Emmenagogue
Rosemary	Abortifacient
Tansy	Abortifacient
Wormwood	Abortifacient

From the first moment we know we are pregnant, we become mothers who want the best for our developing babies. A toxin-free environment in which to grow is our first gift to them. This is why my initial dismay at the lack of 100 percent natural skincare, safe for both mom and baby, inspired the creation of a line of Primal Life Organic Skin-Foods specifically formulated for pregnancy. All our products are guaranteed organic and free of heavy metals, pesticides, and chemicals. Each one is the result of my years of scientific study, extensive research, and a desire to give all children their best first environment. Babies are dependent on the blood flow through the placenta from mom for nourishment, development and growth. Super Power your uterus to provide a healthy home for your current or future growing baby.

Baby Talk

Nature is both amazingly efficient and amazingly complex—and what better example of its complexity than the rapid and constant slew of transformations that occur in an infant's body? Babies grow so fast and change so much that you can practically *see* them growing right before your eyes.

You've already heard me talk about the importance of the skin, and all the functions it performs throughout our lives. Multiply that by 10, and you'll get a sense of the importance and sensitivity of baby skin.

Because of the loose connections between the epidermis and dermis of infant skin, it is much more absorbent than adult skin. Consequently, any product that contacts a baby's skin is much more quickly absorbed than by adults.

Then there's the fact that babies have a greater percentage of body fat than do older children or adults. This means that fat-soluble ingredients in skincare products not only absorb much faster, but also are stored in greater concentrations in all those extra baby fat cells. So what happens when a baby's moisturizer or rash ointment contains additives, stabilizers, colorants, emulsifiers, and fragrances? These ingredients are immediately absorbed and stored away in baby's fat. As a baby grows and becomes leaner, those fat cells diminish and release the stored toxins into the bloodstream, where they can affect damaging neurological changes.

To make matters worse, an infant's ability to manage toxins is much lower than an adult's because the host of chemicals in their environment affects babies more powerfully and more rapidly. And as we've seen, chemicals that are absorbed through the skin do *not* pass through the liver for detoxification and elimination. They first travel to a host of other organs and tissues, and they most definitely make a pit stop in a baby's tiny brain.

Another reason babies face a higher risk of toxicity is that their liver—the main organ responsible for metabolizing these chemicals into water-soluble formulations that can be excreted by the body—is still developing. An immature liver can develop toxic overload, and rashes, allergies, and simple sensitivities may be the first signs of chemical invasion. Unfortunately, these signs are so subtle that they are often overlooked.

All of which explains why assuring your growing infant an environment as free of toxins as possible means giving them a head start on lifelong good health.

Normal baby skin is perfect—soft and elastic, smooth and unblemished. It already contains the natural oils that maintain its luscious creaminess. Washing these oils away with soap means eliminating one barrier of natural protection.

Unless babies fall into a puddle of mud, they rarely need a sudsy, soapy bath. Water alone is sufficient to clean away the sweat, dust, tears, and food that accumulate during normal daily activities.

For messy diapers, I made the Baby's Toilet Water. It contains a small amount of natural cleansers blended into purified water infused with rose, chamomile and green tea. It effectively cleanses the skin without removing natural oils. This helps prevent rashes and breakdown in an area that is often moist and damp. I also applied Baby's Butt Balm as an added protective barrier from the next soiled diaper. I often used Baby's Toilet Water when a quick "bath" was needed. Two or three sprays on a warm washcloth were the easiest bath to give when time was running short.

Baby's Toilet Water is one of my favorite products and I still use it today on my six-year-old and the four-year-old twins. You will find a bottle beside every toilet in my house. During toilet training and even afterward, it is the best product to spray either on the toilet tissue or bum for easy cleaning. It also works great as an underarm freshener, feminine hygiene cleanser, and hand spray (yes, I keep a bottle in my car as well).

But when baby does fall into a puddle of mud, it's important to be certain that the soap you use is not composed of a concentration of chemicals disguised as "gentle" or "natural"—chemicals that a baby's pores suck up in the blink of an eye.

In those cases when real suds are required, I created a Shampoo Bar that works equally well on baby skin and hair. I used it for all three of my children for the occasional times they truly needed more than a simple water bath. All natural and organic, this soap is a cleanser in the purest sense of the word. (That doesn't mean, though, that it won't sting the eyes. You'll still need to take the usual common sense measures to assure that soap doesn't get into a baby's eyes.)

In truth, the hardest thing about maintaining baby's skin may be resisting all the enticing sweet-smelling products on the market for parents of babies. Babies already smell sweet—which is why we grownups can't resist burying our noses in their hair. Unlike all those hyper-scented chemical-laden products Big Cosmo offers, my baby-sensitive products add the smallest possible touch of natural scent to your baby's already wonderful smell.

But what about dryness, diaper rash, breakouts, and other skin irritations? After decades of experience as a nurse and more recently as a mother, I've become convinced that these ailments are usually diet-related. In addition to being susceptible to chemicals, babies are highly vulnerable to allergies to gluten, soy, and dairy. Even some fruits and vegetables can cause minor allergic reactions, but these can come and go, and even be outgrown.

When my babies had the occasional tush rash from dairy or strawberries, I healed it with Baby's Butt Balm or Primal Body Butter. Avoid talc, baby powder, or any other powders—these extreme airway irritants can cause respiratory complications or asthma. Their tiny particles easily disperse in the air, where they can be inhaled into the delicate airway tissue of infants, children, and adults.

A note on improvisation: Use adult-intended products on children sparingly, and be sure to read the labels first. The essential oils in some products for grownups can be too concentrated for sensitive baby skin.

In general, when it comes to skincare for babies and young children, less is more. Less soap means more natural, protective oils in their skin. Babies are already so perfect; we only have to help them stay that way. When you Super Power your uterus, you can't help but Super Power your little one too!

I have the pregnancy version of the Infiniti & Beyond Package with the Ocean face wash. The face wash is amazing—whenever I use it, I feel like it very gently exfoliates dead skin cells without any kind of irritation and my skin is left glowing. The toner is lightweight, and my skin drinks up the serum and especially the moisturizer. Both products just sink right in and feel very nourishing to my face. I really feel that I've got all my bases covered with this set in terms of having a well-rounded skin regimen.

—Marielle

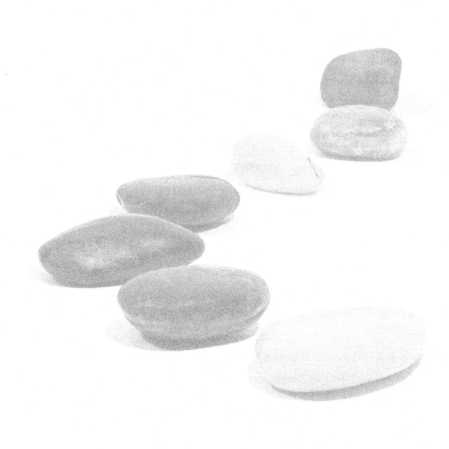

Chapter Nine

Hey, What About MEN?

Please note—this chapter is not just for men. Many women contact me because they are not familiar with skincare and how to use the different products available to maximize their benefits. At the end of this chapter, you will find a "How To" section dedicated to those "minimalists" of both genders who are ready to learn the what, how, and when of a great skincare regime.

Men—sophisticated, affluent, respectable, prized, attractive, and sexy—as much as they might try to deny it, they are concerned with staying that way. Just as women are trying to preserve their youthful appearance, a growing number of men are joining the anti-aging force and arming themselves with their own collection of skincare products.

When I happened to notice the arsenal of beauty and anti-aging products my husband had accumulated, it dawned on me that— until recently—I assumed only women thought moisturizing, deep cleaning, and tightening their skin was critical to their sense of identity.

Not anymore.

I looked at my buff metrosexual husband's lethal slew of face washes, serums, moisturizers, anti-aging facial treatments, and masks in pure amazement. I gazed at his deodorant, toothpaste, shampoo, conditioners, styling gels, cream and sprays, and my jaw dropped. When I got to his body moisturizers, foot lotions, hand lotions, and shaving products, I thought, "I am not the only skin product junkie in this house!"

Humans have a visceral desire, need and drive to look, feel and smell our best. Our skin is a prominent factor in the first impression we make on others. Before we open our mouth, our skin speaks volumes to prospective customers, lovers, neighbors, affiliates, or bosses.

Skincare products are a part of daily living. No matter how off the grid we try to live, for 99 percent of us skincare products are unavoidable. When I started my company, my target audience was primarily women. But this has changed. Today Primals of both genders desire the same thing—lasting beauty and health.

But at what cost? What is the true cost of looking good—not just the pocketbook cost but the long-term *health cost*? Is it worth it to look good today or pay less for a product today, only to suffer the health consequences in the future?

Men are just as interested as women in getting the POWER back. Going back to what nature offers. Healing the body towards anti-aging instead of chemically altering the cells. Big Cosmo duped men just as well as they duped women. Men clearly want to look and feel good, young, and attractive just as much as women. Big Cosmo knows this and has capitalized on this reality.

However, we are heading toward a culture of INDEPENDENCE. We want control over our health and we want the power to choose what goes in and on our bodies. We are changing the way we view skincare. It's no longer just a necessity to look and feel better; it's a long-term investment into our health—for both men and women.

Surprisingly, there is little difference between the needs of a man's skin versus that of a woman's. We are both covered in the same outer coating, though they may function in slightly different ways. Other than the fact that men grow facial hair and most women don't, what are the unique properties of men's skin that makes it differ from women's?

Men have a predominance of testosterone (androgen) that causes an increase in the epidural thickness of their skin; it can be up to 25 percent thicker than a woman's. Due to this thicker epidural layer, men's skin is rougher and has larger pores that clog more easily from dirt and oil.

Men's skin tends to have a higher collagen density than women's. Collagen is a strengthening protein that women lose at a faster rate than men. It has been said that a woman's skin is about 15 years older than a man's of her same age.

Whether it's thick or dry, all skin needs moisture. After puberty, men produce more sebum than women. Sebum is made by the sebaceous glands. They exist in every part of our body except on hands and feet, but are most concentrated in the forehead and chin. The sebum they produce moisturizes the skin. Testosterone increases this oil production, which could be why men tend to have longer-lasting acne issues, especially during puberty. Estrogen, on the other hand, tends to diminish oil production—a reason why women tend to have dry, flaky skin.

What it boils down to is this: Both men and women need oils and essential oils for complete skin nourishment and hydration. Oils and essential oils are the perfect diet for facial skin because they contain omegas, vitamins, essential fatty acids, antioxidants, and more. Women's thinner skin will tend to absorb the oils within 15 minutes. Men's thicker skin may require a little more volume and may take slightly longer to fully absorb. But that's also the reason why men need to exfoliate.

And here's why:

Shaving facial hair every day further dehydrates and damages the skin. Not to mention that all commercial shaving creams, lotions, and gels contain harmful ingredients that assault skin that's just been scraped with a razor, leaving easy entry for toxins.

Increasing evidence shows that damage to sperm production; male genital abnormalities in newborn boys, and growing rates of male prostate and breast cancers are linked to endocrine disruptors in the thousands of chemicals polluting our lives. In our skincare products, many of these ingredients act as weak estrogen that negatively affects young, developing males when they are most sensitive to it.

Every health concern I have discussed in this book affects every human from conception through death. Men are no exception to the list. Cancers, hormone disrupters, Alzheimer's disease, concentration problems, irritable bowel syndrome, bloating, leaky gut, slowed metabolism, and even infertility are not gender or age specific. Using all natural, organic skincare products is important for our beauty but critical for our health.

I married a metrosexual man, and LOVE that about him. He isn't vain—he is health conscious and as interested in maintaining his healthy outer appearance as many women are. Contrasting him, I am a minimalist when it comes to beauty products—I like it plain and simple. Josh is familiar with all levels of skincare, has exceptional insight, and is typically the first tester (outside of staff) of our new products. His main concern with Big-Cosmo skincare products is that they contain endocrine and hormone disrupters.

Many of the chemicals (especially those questionable undisclosed chemicals in colognes and perfumes) have been linked to a lowered sperm count. Prostate cancer is on the rise, and should be a concern for the entire male population, just as breast cancer should be a concern for all women. If the ingredients in commercial deodorant are showing up in the lumps and tumors from breast tissue, what are they doing to the prostate? The hormone-disrupting elements have been linked with prostate cancer as well as infertility. Speaking of breast cancer, another interesting fact (as a nurse anesthetist I witnesses this routinely) is that breast cancer also affects men, and is on the rise.

Because my products are free of toxins, my husband enjoys using almost all of them, and I love having his male perspective. The only products he hasn't tested are the Primal Hair products, only because he is shaved bald. But even that has been a great testing ground for his novel use of our other products. He discovered that using Dirty Ex Sweet Revenge—an oil/sugar exfoliator—on his head before he shaves gives him a much smoother and closer shave. And he likes to brag about how soft his head feels!

I think the biggest turn-off for men and skincare is the fact that most commercial products are geared toward women and "fragranced" that way. Let's face it—most men don't want to smell like a rose! None of the my creations have offended or threatened my husband's manly scent—including Primal PitStick in lavender. Yes, Josh even tested this scent for himself and wore it at his CrossFit Akron box.

In a way—because they typically use unscented products—men's resistance to smelling like flowers has prevented their absorption of many of the destructive neurotoxins in fragrances. And their skin and organs may be in better shape because of it, too.

As the years pass, more and more men ask me about the products they use on their skin. Often they don't know where or how to begin, what to purchase, how to use all the products, and what it all means.

Most men use soap to wash and maybe a little moisturizer. They don't use toners, serums, treatments, and makeup. Until recently, many men weren't really sure what toner is, how to moisturize, when to wash, what direction to apply eye serum, and where to exfoliate. But this is changing quickly.

Most men really do want to look their best and will put in the effort when they understand the how, what, and when. But they often don't want to ask. Take heart, Great Adventurers into the beauty products world—you are not alone.

Start slow and keep it simple. See how your skin reacts to the added nutrients. Listen to your skin. It will tell you what it loves and what it can do without.

Begin, for instance, with a simple face wash (Bare Primal Face Wash is perfect for all skin types and offers a gentle conversion to toxin-free skincare). You may wish to add the exfoliating scrub that Josh uses: Dirty Ex Sweet Revenge. You'll notice the smoothness of your skin and the tingle of increased circulation after only one application. When you're comfortable with that, you may want to add the Bare Primal Face Moisturizer to help protect against aging and the elements.

Let curiosity guide you toward other products or you can write to me at support@PrimalLifeOrganics.com with any questions you have.

No matter what products you choose or who you buy from, always read, read, read your labels! Using freshly made and nutrient dense real-food products from Primal Organics means you have a guarantee that you will be able to pronounce every ingredient on the label. Buy from a company that cares about your long-term health. Skip the preservatives and extended shelf life.

Take control back. Let your skin speak to you. Learn how to listen to your skin. Wash away the chemical trance, detox your cells and see how real foods lead to radiant skin.

No matter where you start or how extensive your skincare regimen, truly natural skincare is a straight shot to good health and wickedly good-looking skin.

A STEP-BY-STEP GUIDE
FOR THE (MALE) MINIMALIST

Being a skincare minimalist has its advantages for both genders. Treating your skin to some added nutrients definitely will give it more vitality and youthfulness. These directions are for Primal Life Organics Primal Face Wash, Toner, Moisturizers, Serums, Exfoliators, and Face Masks. If you use a different brand, please remember to read your labels carefully because the directions may be different.

1. CLEANSER

Clean skin is like a clean canvas. It functions best when it can breathe because skin not only absorbs what is applied; it also expels what is metabolized (waste products). Remember, as a man your pores are larger and more easily clogged with oils and dirt. Congested skin pores lead to irritation, rashes, melasma (brown discoloration), and acne.

During sleep, the body heals, repairs and expels waste. Washing in the morning freshens the skin and removes whatever was expelled during the night. Be careful to wash with a gentle cleanser. Harsh chemicals like sodium lauryl sulfate strip away the layer of protective oils your skin creates—and along with this protective layer goes your body's first line of defense.

The sebum that moisturizes the skin contains medium-chain triglycerides (MCTs). Your skin surface harbors protective bacteria that live synergistically with you. It is estimated that the number of bacteria living in and on the human body outnumbers the body's internal cells 10 to 1. These lipophilic microbes (natural surface bacteria) consume the glycol portion of the MCT and leave behind medium-chain fatty acids (MCFA). These MCFA kill pathogenic bacteria, virus, and fungi. Commercial soaps strip away these natural defenders, but Primal Organics face washes cleanse the surface of your skin yet leaves the protective layer intact. Your skin won't have that tight, dry feeling because you get to keep your MCFAs.

Wash or cleanse your skin in the morning and before bed.

Primal Face Wash: Gently shake the bottle, then wet hands. Apply half a dropper-full (approximately 10–15 drops) onto damp hands and rub together. Massage the sudsy lather onto your face. Rinse with warm water. PAT DRY with a soft towel. Even though your skin is thick, rubbing it with a towel causes micro tears in your skin and capillaries—exactly what we try to avoid as we age.

2. TONER

Toners are a combination of moisturizers, oils, and extracts. They all help soothe your skin in different ways, and help maintain its pH balance so your moisturizer will absorb better. AVOID astringents—they contain alcohol that tightens the skin, pulls the moisture out of it, and dehydrates your cells.

Primal Face Toner: Gently shake then lightly spray 3–4 pumps on your clean, dry facial and neck skin. Let dry for 30–60 seconds.

3. SERUM OR MOISTURIZER

Men need moisture just as much as women, and sometimes even more. If your moisturizer is made from real food sources and is organic, it adds nutrients and oils to your skin. Obviously, well-nourished skin cells function better than dehydrated and starving ones.

Most commercial moisturizers are primarily water, and we now know why water actually dries out the skin rather than hydrating it. Consequently, when people first begin using any Primal Life Organics product, they use way too much. Normally, people use two to four times the amount of our product than they need. Why? Because our serums and moisturizers are water-free and nutrient dense, so a very small amount goes a very long way.

Start with just a little. The next time, use even less and keep reducing the amount you use until you've found the perfect small amount that is right for you.

Primal Face Serum: Apply one drop to cheeks, forehead, and chin. Massage gently.

Primal Face Moisturizer: Scoop a small amount from jar and gently massage into skin.

Both the serum and moisturizer can be used on the sensitive skin under your eyes. Just be sure to apply *very gently* and *in the direction from outer eye to inner eye.* Using the outer-to-inner motion will help prevent damage to that very delicate tissue under your eyes.

This easy three-step plan will give your skin a daily dose of everything it needs to look fresh and function well.

There is no real need to use both a serum and moisturizer unless you feel your skin needs the extra moisture. On days when you spend hours in the sun, wind, or dirt, you may want to apply both, 20 minutes apart. On normal days, one or the other is plenty. Listen to your skin: it will tell you what it wants.

Now let's look at a couple of awesome ways to deep clean and nourish your skin. These are my favorite skincare luxury treatments, and you can use them once or twice a week.

EXFOLIATORS

New skin cells are constantly rising to the surface and old ones need to be removed. As we age this process of cell turnover slows down, cells pile up unevenly on the skin's surface, clog pores, and make your skin look dry, rough, and dull.

Always based on some sort of "rough" ingredient (sand, coffee grounds, almond meal, sugar, salt, or apricot seeds), exfoliators are massaged onto the face to remove dead skin cells and excess buildup. Afterward, your skin feels and looks vibrant and strong because you've just stimulated the circulation, revealed the younger skin cells, and given it a dose of delicious nutrients.

Primal Life Organics offers two facial exfoliators—Dirty Ex @ Midnight and Dirty Ex Sweet Revenge. One is a powder and the other is an oil/sugar scrub. Both are so refreshing that you risk becoming an exfoliant addict.

Freshly exfoliated skin absorbs nutrients better, so this is my favorite time to use a face treatment serum that packs a punch!

FIRE AND ICE TREATMENT SYSTEM is a two-step process that combines the heat of cayenne pepper with the cooling sensation of menthol crystals to increase blood flow and decongest the skin.

Step 1: FIRE

Fire Serum is made from cayenne pepper infused into jojoba oil. Why cayenne? Because it is high in vitamins A, B complex, C, calcium, and potassium. Did you know that cayenne reduces pain and inflammation? The capsicum in cayenne is the ingredient that makes the peppers hot, but it also has mild antibacterial properties, which can destroy some of the bacteria that cause acne.

Added to Fire are three essential oils (palmarosa, Peru balsam, and petitgrain), all of which are superior in their decongestant properties. These oils nourish, soothe, and smooth dry skin and diminish wrinkles. They also stimulate cell regeneration for more youthful skin.

Fire Serum is a powerful formula that's best used at night. Avoid getting it in your eyes or too close to your mouth. If you do, it'll sting for about 20 minutes (trust me, I know from experience!), but will not cause any damage.

How to use it: Apply one drop to cheeks, forehead, and chin. Gently massage. Allow your skin to absorb it for about 20 minutes. You'll feel the heat as the capsicum is absorbed. The sensation can get a little intense for about 15 minutes. I *love* this sensation—I know the serum is working and bringing my senses alive!

DO NOT RINSE OFF—APPLY ICE SERUM DIRECTLY ON TOP OF FIRE SERUM.

Step 2: ICE

Ice contains menthol crystals that do more than just diminish the heat from Fire Serum. The menthol will activate your skin's cold receptors and cause a cooling sensation that soothes irritation of swollen or inflamed tissues and reduces pain, swelling, and tenderness. It also re-balances natural oil production.

Ice contains numerous oils and essential oils that nourish and moisturize facial cells in an intense, targeted way. It's packed with powerful antioxidants that neutralize those free radicals that damage skin and cause aging.

These same nutrients help increase collagen, skin strength and elasticity, and deliver high levels of omegas and vitamins A, B-1, B-2, B-3, D, E, and F. Vitamins A and F are actively involved in the rejuvenation and renewal of cell membranes. Vitamin E is a superior antioxidant that fights free radical damage and prevents aging. Omegas-3, -6, and -9 in baobab oil improve skin elasticity, encourage regeneration of skin cells and epithelial tissue, and improve skin tone. Ice also contains foods that help diminish scars left by acne as well as fades discolorations and age spots by promoting new cell growth.

And what better time to deliver this feast of nutrients than when the blood flow is already generously increased by your Fire Serum treatment? This means better absorption and utilization of all the nutrients!

How to use it: Twenty minutes after applying Fire Serum, apply Ice in the same way—a drop to forehead, both cheeks, and chin. Be sure to avoid eyes and mouth because residual Fire will mix with Ice. Massage it in gently. When you use Fire and Ice, you can skip your normal moisturizer if desired.

DO NOT RINSE OFF. Go to bed and let sleep regenerate your body while Fire and Ice rejuvenate your skin.

FIRE AND ICE TREATMENT is the ultimate skin-food home treatment to give you spa-grade effects. Your face will tingle from the warmth of cayenne plus the high contrast of cooling menthol.

It is the perfect balance of hot and cold reduces and reverses damage from the elements and the aging process. Not only will your skin be fed incredible nutrients, but also your senses will come alive along with it!

FACE MASKS

Giving yourself a facial mask has to be one of life's little pleasures. Giving yourself a facial mask that also packs in a powerhouse of nutrients means more bang for your buck.

Primal Life Organics Face Masks are made with our motto in mind: natural, fresh, and pure. And they are made from Mother Nature's finest secrets: clays, herbs, and food sources.

Our Face Masks heal, nourish, hydrate, and support skin functions. They facilitate detoxification, draw out impurities, calm, soothe, and rejuvenate. They exfoliate dead cells and reveal new, youthful ones. They're beneficial for any skin type and come in many forms, shapes, and sizes.

How to use it: Take a small amount of the powder and mix it with a small amount of water, just enough to make mud (I mix this in the palm of my hand). Apply the mud to your face, avoiding your eyes and mouth. Let it dry for 5–10 minutes. The tightening you feel is the drawing out of toxins and excess oils from your pores. Afterward, rinse with water.

Your skin will look and feel great—refreshed, soft, nourished, and detoxified.

PUTTING IT ALL TOGETHER:

Here's a step-by-step cheat sheet of daily and weekly treatments for your optimum skin care routine.

TREATMENT	DAILY	WEEKLY
1. Wash	✓	✓
2. Exfoliate		✓
3. Face Mask		✓
4. Toner	✓	✓
5. Fire and Ice		✓
6. Serum or Moisturizer	✓	

Your skin is the organ that mirrors your inner vitality. Treat it well, feed it well, and it will reward you!

_____

I am so amazed with this Banished Primal Blemish Serum. I have tried every product out there. When I shave, I get tiny bumps around my mouth and chin area. I use Banished Primal Blemish Serum after shaving and the bumps are gone by morning! This stuff is the BEST!! And I LOVE the tingle—I know it's working!

—*Alex*

CHAPTER TEN

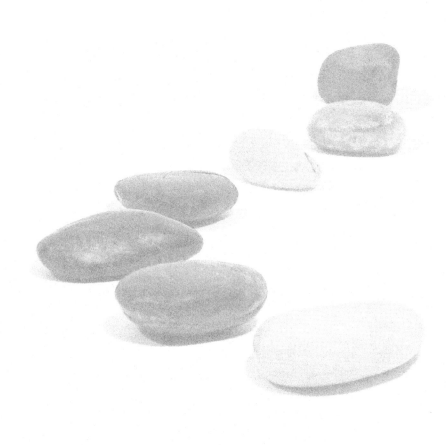

Diet: How to Super Power Your Skin

I created my skincare so I could have toxic-free, radiant, glowing skin. I created Primal Life Organics so you can, too!
—Trina Felber, CEO Primal Life Organics RN, BSN, MSN, CRNA

There are hundreds of organic skincare companies out there, so why choose Primal Life Organics? What sets us apart from all of the others?

I have Super Powered my skin. I created Primal Life Organics to help you Super Power your skin. I know what it takes. I know how it feels. I know where you are, where you are heading, and how you can make the change. It's not difficult to Super Power your skin, but it does take commitment. It's only three simple steps. Ditch the chemicals. Detox your cells. Feed your skin real-food. I provide the food to heal your body.

Approximately 95 percent of skincare companies use ingredients that harm the body. The other 5 percent provide true organic, natural skincare. But being organic is no assurance that the product doesn't contain contaminants—it only means the main ingredients were grown without chemicals or hormones. A product can be organic but still contain health-harming chemicals that make that product long lasting or sudsy or sweet smelling.

Primal Life Organics goes above and beyond the top 5 percent by using organic ingredients *and* making our products fresh to order. And we *never* use chemicals, in any form. My endeavors are your body's pleasures. Delicious for your body and your skin.

On our shelves there are no products, only ingredients. They are primal, in their natural state. Just like our ancestors looked to nature for their body care and rubbed pure oils on their skin, Primal Life Organics uses the simplest form of each pure ingredient in order to reap the greatest amount of its benefits. Our organic ingredients are just waiting to be custom-made into your order to ensure your skin, body, organs, tissues, and cells receive the highest quality nutrition available.

This is the MY Guarantee:

Quality — Freshness — Results

> ❯ Our Skin-Food is made in a kitchen, not a factory!

> ❯ Our Skin-Food is made by humans, not machines.

> ❯ Our kitchen does NOT contain any gluten, toxins, artificial fragrances, chemicals or preservatives—just food, dirt, and plants.

> ❯ Our Skin-Food is made fresh when ordered, and guarantees a nutrient-dense product, not a nutrient-deprived one.

> Our Skin-Food heals, nourishes, protects, and gives results—safely.

> Our Skin-Food is so real you can eat it! Bon Appétit!

Nature had it right. Think about it. Before labs were invented, we looked to the soil to produce our food and nutrition. We used dirt to cleanse, brush our teeth, wash our hair and detoxify our day away. We used plants to provide the micro nutrients to heal, protect and soothe. We made oils, tinctures and extract to treat ailments and conditions. Before Big Cosmo brain washed us and contaminated our nervous system, we knew what we knew… and we knew nature was all we needed for youth, vitality, energy, detox, healing, protection and power.

I built my company on these principles. Getting back to nature—the primal life—is the way to heal, protect and nourish. Food is delicious for my body and my skin. My skin has never looked better. I'm done with the empty promises Big Cosmo offers. Sick from their chemicals. Now that I have detoxed and dose my skin daily with real nutrients, my skin speaks to me. My skin loves me back. My skin is radiant and glowing. I have Super Power Skin. I know Beauty's Dirty Secret. I live in harmony with Mother Nature.

Natural beauty comes from nature. Nature is vibrant, alive, tough, free, toned, energetic, oxygenated, and forgiving. What comes from nature breeds life. Food breeds life. Food provides the energy for cells to sustain life. Without proper food, cells die. With proper food, they thrive.

Primal Life Organics is synonymous with REAL food for your skin. That's why we call our products "Skin-Food." We provide the food that keeps your cells vibrant, alive, tough, free, toned, energetic, oxygenated, and forgiving. Real food heals the body. Well-fed skin is radiant and glowing.

My products work synergistically with the cells. Cells that are fed real food can handle stress. When toxins enter the body, they are easily metabolized into water-soluble compounds and excreted by the urine, gastrointestinal tract, respiratory system, or skin.

Cells that function properly easily recover when compromised. Antioxidants easily disarm free radicals and allow your body to work at its optimum. Your brain is clear, your energy is high, and your skin is glowing.

Four Benefits to Ordering Skincare Products from a Real Food Skincare Company

There are myriad benefits to ordering your health and skincare products from an organic, real food skincare company. If you're new to the world of organic skincare, here are four easy reasons why *your* next purchase should be not just organic, but from a skincare company with nutrient-dense products, like Primal Life Organics:

1. Free of toxins, chemicals and artificial ingredients

The number one reason to make the switch to organic real food skincare products is to provide your skin—your body's first defense against toxins and disease—with pure, natural, and safe treatment. Organic real food products use recognizable foods like beeswax, fruits and vegetables, animal and nut oils, and seaweed, plus essential oils, salt, and clay to craft products your body recognizes and can fully use. Not one of these products was pumped up, damped down, or otherwise twisted by chemical enhancers, preservatives, colorants, etc.

2. Orders made fresh for each customer

At Primal Life Organics the shelves are stocked with *ingredients*, not products. To give you the highest quality product, we create your order with fresh, natural ingredients. That is why we don't need preservatives or fillers, and why you won't find a "super size" in our product line. We package our products in sizes that match a typical rate of consumption, so you always have freshness on your skin and on your side.

3. Consistent with Vegan, Paleo, and Gluten-free lifestyles

We make sure all of our ingredients have a relationship with dirt and are from *real food* sources, but don't encourage adverse reactions from that number one allergen—gluten. If you're committed to putting only quality ingredients *in* your body, it just makes sense that you should only put the same quality *on* your body.

4. Improves skin tone and quality

One of the greatest benefits of organic, *real food* skincare products is the profound difference you'll see in your skin. The color, tone, and texture of your skin will improve through the use of skincare products free of harsh chemicals and other irritants and rich in vitamins, minerals, and essential fatty acids in forms the body understands, requires and can use.

Where to Start?

It is overwhelming to look at our skincare needs and discover just how many products we use every day! *Some products we use twice a day!* So where do you start? What do you change first?

I believe in starting with the basics, so I created a Starter Package as an introduction to 100% natural skin and body care that will help facilitate a smooth transition into chemical free and natural skincare. It is the perfect way to try out a selection of our bestselling facial, dental and body products. Feeding your skin the basic building blocks of nutrition from real food sources that your skin can utilize immediately will deliver the best results. Things you use every day can cause more harm than good, so I recommend starting with your deodorant (or antiperspirant) and your toothpaste.

As we said in Chapter Four, both of these products contain numerous ingredients that harm your body. Since both of these products are daily staples in most skincare routines, let's take a closer look at how and why going toxic-free with both of these can drastically improve your health.

I believe in preventing disease. The best way to prevent disease is by ensuring that our cells are healthy.

When we use deodorant, our goal is to prevent offensive body odor. Using commercial deodorant or antiperspirant does the trick.

The danger here is you are also allowing chemicals into your body that are associated with cancer, Alzheimer's disease, endocrine disruption, reproductive disorders, and more. These chemicals have also been implicated in breast tumors, but there are conflicting reports as to whether the specific chemicals in deodorants are the actual cause of the tumor.

Research shows that the aluminum prevents sweating. But when you stop the sweating process, toxins are not released (as intended) through your sweat glands. Instead they travel via the lymph system to other organs where they can cause cancer. Aluminum from antiperspirants has also been found in the brains of people with Alzheimer's disease. Given the frightening rates of this dread disease in modern society[15], it seems only logical to eliminate one possible cause of it by changing to a deodorant that is free of aluminum.

I am not debating the truth of any of this. My point is this: If there is any possibility of harm that is reason enough to find a better solution.

My solution to conventional deodorant/antiperspirant is the Primal Life Organics Stick Up Deodorant. Since it is not an antiperspirant, it allows you to sweat: healthfully and naturally purging toxins from your body. The Stick Up works by inhibiting the growth of bacteria, which is what causes odor.

When you first make the switch to the Stick Up (or any natural deodorant) you may experience increased sweating and odor. Remember detox? If not, reread Chapter Five. This is what is happening.

This detox may occur for up to six weeks while your body rids itself of the toxins that are stored in the body fat. Secondly, your body needs to adjust to this change, especially if you used an antiperspirant to prevent sweating. Releasing the toxins will help cleanse your body and the amount you sweat will decrease with time.

---

15 http://www.alz.org/alzheimers_disease_facts_and_figures.asp#quickFacts

During the first few weeks using the Stick Up, you may need to reapply two or three times a day. When you notice an odor, just reapply the Stick Up and it will take the odor away. Soon, you should be able to apply just once a day.

What's Wrong with My Toothpaste?

Most commercial toothpastes contain at least three potentially harmful—possibly toxic—and unnecessary chemicals: glycerin, sodium lauryl sulfate (SLS), and artificial sweeteners. Fluoride—which many people avoid because of its toxicity—is also common in commercial mouth care.

What most consumers don't realize is that these chemicals actually *weaken* the enamel and cause the minerals that strengthen the teeth to leech out of the teeth instead (demineralization). A weakened tooth is very susceptible to the elements, sugars, and chemicals. Once breakdown occurs, cavities result.

A look at the most common and destructive chemicals:

Glycerin is thought to leave a coating on the teeth, possibly contributing to de-mineralization and preventing re-mineralization (the layering of minerals on the enamel to strengthen and protect the tooth).

Sodium lauryl sulfate (SLS) is readily absorbed by the body and considered a "probable human carcinogen" by the Environmental Working Group (EWG). According to the EWG, SLS may cause skin irritation, eye irritation, and even hormone imbalances. Exposure may also cause denaturing of structural protein, including the membranes in our mouths. A review of the available literature on SLS by the National Industrial Chemicals Notification and Assessment Scheme[16] indicated eye and skin irritation as clinically observed.

SLS and Sodium Lauroyl Sarcosinate are synthetic chemicals used as foaming agents in toothpaste (see chemical chart on page 56). SLS is commonly found in engine degreaser, garage floor cleaners, and car wash soaps[17]. In the scientific community, it is a known skin irritant linked to mouth ulcers and canker sores[18].

Commercial products often include a variety of *artificial sweeteners* intended to make them palatable.

Saccharine, one of the most common, is manufactured from petroleum products. And like most artificial sweeteners, it has been linked to cancer.[19]

Sorbitol and **aspartame** are two other common artificial sweeteners. The possible side effects of these chemicals is *scary*: headaches, dizziness, mood changes, vomiting or nausea, abdominal pain/cramps, change in vision, diarrhea, seizures/convulsions, memory loss, fatigue, numbness in legs, joint pain, unexplainable depression, anxiety attacks, slurred speech, blurred vision, multiple sclerosis, fibromyalgia, systemic lupus, and various cancers.[20] Many of these side effects are surprisingly common. People suffer from them, but it's very difficult to link the symptoms their chemical cause.

16 nicnas.gov.au
17 http://dherbs.com/articles/beware-of-toothpaste-222.html
18 http://voices.yahoo.com/fluoride-other-hidden-toxins-toothpaste-70307.html?cat=5
19 http://www.ewg.org/search/site/saccharine%20and%20cancer
20 http://www.medicinenet.com/artificial_sweeteners/page8.htm#aspartamecon

Aspartame is the chemical name for the brand names Nutra-Sweet, Equal, Spoonful, and Equal-Measure. It is made up of three chemicals: aspartic acid, phenylalanine, and methanol. Did you know that a by-product of aspartame is *formaldehyde?* For a great article on the dangers of aspartame, read the article, "Aspartame is, by Far, the Most Dangerous Substance on the Market that is Added To Foods."[21]

All of you gum chewers, diet pop drinkers, diet yogurt eaters, and consumers of "diet" and "sugar-free" anything—PAY ATTEN-TION! Aspartame is used in almost all "sugar-free" and "diet" substances.

Fluoride has actually been categorized as a "toxic drug" by the FDA[22]. If you are buying organic food to avoid pesticides but using commercial toothpaste, you might be interested to know that sodium fluoride was at one time widely used as an *insecticide and a rodenticide (rodent killer)*[23].

Fluoride toxicity from toothpaste can happen with chronic fluoride exposure just by taking in a little with every brushing. It can have harmful effects throughout the entire body.

Fluoride can cause dental fluorosis—enamel discoloration from damage to the tooth-forming cells—in children. Studies show that fluoride causes brain damage, possibly causing IQ deficits in children. It can also adversely affect the pineal gland, thyroid gland, bones, and gastrointestinal tract. And it has been linked to bone and bladder cancers.

Now, think of your kids. Do you think that, on occasion, they swallow some of the toothpaste you put on their brushes? Maybe even you do sometimes? And even if you're not swallowing it, you

21 http://articles.mercola.com/sites/articles/archive/2011/11/06/aspartame-most-dangerous-substance-added-to-food.aspx
22 http://downwithbasics.com/the-5-hidden-dangers-in-toothpaste
23 http://downwithbasics.com/the-5-hidden-dangers-in-toothpaste

are still putting it into your mouth where it has access to the rest of your body via sublingual absorption. Is that a risk you are willing to put on yourself and your family?

Concerns over toxic or harsh ingredients may seem overblown until you think about this: if you brush your teeth for two minutes, twice a day, your gums are exposed to the toothpaste for a full 24 hours each year! In the long run, every second counts, so using a paste that is nontoxic and free of industrially formulated chemicals is critical. Why take a 24-hour chemical bath every year?

What about brushing? You've probably heard that hand washing should last at least two minutes for maximum effectiveness. Just like washing your hands, brushing for two minutes is actually as important **as the products you use. If you can't find** good toothpaste, you can simply use water. In fact, the simple act of BRUSHING for two minutes is likely more effective at cleaning your teeth than conventional toothpaste![24]

Teeth are equated to living stone—they are living, porous material that requires minerals to remain strong. These minerals MUST come in contact with the demineralized spot on the tooth's surface or re-mineralization will not occur. You cannot take a supplement or vitamin internally. Re-mineralization must occur inside the mouth. Furthermore, because the Standard American Diet is lacking in the minerals the teeth need to stay strong, the chemical reaction that should take place within the mouth to convert the minerals from the food into the mineral ions the teeth can absorb, does not happen. As a result, the teeth loose the minerals, sensitivities develop as a sign of demineralization, and if the minerals are not replaced, cavities develop. Primal Life Organics Dirty Mouth Toothpowder is made from direct-from-the-earth ingredients, no laboratory required.

---

24 http://www.livestrong.com/article/260192-the-best-ways-to-water-clean-teeth/

Dirty Mouth Toothpowder contains three different clays. The clays contain the mineral ions needed by the teeth to re-mineralize and remain strong. If the teeth are lacking the minerals, and there are holes in the latticework of the enamel, the mineral ions from the clays are in direct contact with the surface of the weakened enamel and can be absorbed into the enamel for re-mineralization. Teeth can and do heal, but only if the minerals are in the correct form and in direct contact with the teeth.

Our toothpowder provides protection from plaque and cavities, delivers nutrients for healthy gums and teeth, and is toxin-free. It provides essential minerals that are absorbed through gum tissue and porous teeth.[25] It whitens and cleans with *gently* abrasive earthen clays, and leaves the delicate oral tissues feeling fresh.

Many native cultures with robust dental health practice oral hygiene that is unfamiliar to us, but we can certainly learn from them. The practice of "pica"—the ingestion of dirt or clay—is common among tribal communities. Pica is the body compelling us to obtain minerals that are lacking in the diet.

I'm not suggesting you eat a bowl of dirt for dinner, but knowing that traditional cultures value clay for its mineral density, and understanding how critical minerals are to the health of the mouth (nutrition for the teeth), using clay for dental health and re-mineralization just makes sense.

The chemicals in commercial toothpaste can actually leech the minerals from the teeth, causing a weak and brittle surface that is more prone to damage and decay.

---

25 Stoeken, Judith; Spiros, Paraskevas; van der Weijden, Godefridus A., *The Long-Term Effect of a Mouthrinse Containing Essential Oils on Dental Plaque and Gingivitis: A Systematic Review*, Journal of Periodontology Jul 2007, Vol. 78, No. 7, Pages 1218-1228

With continued use of Dirty Mouth Toothpowder, your teeth get stronger because our toothpowder promotes enamel re-mineralization. The minerals in our toothpowder are the minerals your teeth need to maintain integrity and strength, and to fight cavities.

Breaking Your Bad Habit

I am a nurse, but long after I graduated from school and got my MS in Nursing, I still had a bad habit, one that you probably have, too. It made me sick, bloated, tired, forgetful, fat, and lazy. My skin was dull and broken out and oily.

What was my destructive habit? I never read my product labels!

By not knowing what was in my skincare products, I didn't know I was poisoning myself with chemicals or that they were responsible for my constant acne, oily skin, and recurrent bloating. I didn't know that the toxic ingredients in my "natural" or high-end products were attacking my immune system, creating inflammation in my body, and promoting disease. Changing your habits is the hardest thing you may face during your switch from a life filled with toxins to one filled with health-promoting nutrients.

But most of what you do every single day is done by habit. Getting out of bed and heading to the bathroom, making breakfast, driving to work—so habitual, you may not realize you are doing them. Habits are actions repeated so much they are automatic. They develop over time because you need to take care of yourself.

Most of us buy our skincare products the same way. We know right where they are in the store, so we automatically head to that spot. We automatically choose the exact shelf they sit on and quickly scan for the package we expect to find. Then we take them home and automatically put them in their reserved place in our shelves. Later, we automatically reach for the bottle, smell the fragrance, and feel the texture.

Not once do we read the label and know what our habitual purchases contain.

Break that bad habit of always being on automatic! Become aware of your choices. Replace your bad habit with a good practice until it's your new, best habit: READ THE LABELS.

Set yourself up for success and health.

Throughout this book, you've learned about Big Cosmo's dirty and deceptive secrets. I've shared the dirty secrets of Mother Nature as well, but her secrets are of pure intention. You've learned how and why commercial products damage your body, promote the very problems they profess to cure, and diminish your health.

Now you also have a guide to freeing your skin and body—and your family's—from these negative impacts. Starting with pregnancy and continuing through all life stages, you can rest easy knowing that I am 100 percent on your side, preserving and promoting the good health that is the foundation of living life long, in the best ways possible.

Read all of your labels and make one change at a time. I am here for you. I will help in any way that I can. You can contact me at support@primallifeorganics.com with any questions, concerns, or thoughts.

I wish you happy cells, shining skin, and a strong body that looks its best. Stop the skin war. Remember, the choice is yours. Knowledge is power. Take the power back and take control of your body and skin. Don't let Big Cosmo keep you in a chemical trance. Now you know Beauty's Dirty Secret. Break free. Super Power Your Skin. Ditch the chemicals. Detox your body. Feed your skin real food. Purify and experience what your skin really feels like. The Great Skin Lie has just been uncovered.

THE GREAT SKIN TRUTH
PRIMAL LIFE ORGANICS

Primal Life Organics offers you over 100 products to complement your life and your health at any age:

BODY

Skincare products made for the whole body and created with the best natural oils, essential oils, herbs, foods, clays, salts, and sugars:

1. Blossom Belly Serum
2. Cindy's Primal WOD Package
3. Diane's Primal WOD Package
4. Fran's Primal WOD Package
5. Stick Up, 100% Natural Deodorant
6. Funki Primal Foot Repair
7. Primal Body Butter *
8. Primal Body Butter, Fallen
9. Primal Face and Body Package *
10. Primal Hand Repair, Unscented
11. Sun-Up & Sun-Down Package *
12. Sun-Down After Sun Moisturizer
13. Sun-Up Before Sun Protector
14. Torn Up Primal Skin Repair

FACE

Banished and Beyond *products specially designed for acne-prone skin and that provide the ultimate Skin-Food to nourish, heal, repair, and revitalize your skin to minimize new scars and help fade existing scars and discolorations due to acne:*

1. Banished and Beyond Package for Acne *
2. Banished Primal Blemish Serum *
3. Banished Primal Face Mask for Acne *
4. Banished Primal Face Toner
5. Banished Primal Face Wash
6. Banished Primal Face Moisturizer

Bare *products contain natural oils that heal, moisturize, nourish, and help prevent aging for all skin types:*

1. Bare Primal Face Package
2. Bare Primal Face Wash
3. Bare Face Moisturizer

Beyond *products contain premium natural ingredients that help diminish signs of aging, fade acne scars and discolorations, reduce fine lines and wrinkles, improve skin color, tone, and texture as well as speed cellular regeneration:*

1. Beyond Primal Face Moisturizer
2. Beyond Primal Face Serum

Carrot Seed Line *is specifically formulated for oily skin to help normalize sebum production and improve cellular regeneration:*

1. Carrot Seed Primal Face Moisturizer
2. Carrot Seed Primal Face Package, Norm-Oily
3. Carrot Seed Primal Face Serum
4. Carrot Seed Primal Face Wash

Dirty Ex products *are facial exfoliators made with detoxifying clays to help exfoliate the skin and remove impurities*

1. Dirty Ex Midnight
2. Dirty Ex Package
3. Dirty Ex Sweet Revenge

Other facial products designed with your health and good looks in mind:

1. Earth Primal Face Wash—made with oils, earthen clays, and herbs
2. Ocean Primal Face Wash, Aging Skin—made with oils, dulse seaweed, and Himalayan sea salt
3. Primal Herbal-Clay Face Mask Anti-Aging—clarifying face mask made from clays and herbs that prevents aging by improving skin tone, texture, and clarity
4. Fire and Ice, Primal Face Treatment—two-step facial treatment system to detoxify skin and improve color, tone, and texture as well as fade scars and discoloration

5. Grunt Primal Lip Balm *—moisturizing lip balm that protects, soothes, and softens lips

6. Harmony Primal Face Moisturizer—for all skin types

Infiniti Line products *are designed to prevent and reduce signs of aging, and can be alternated with the* Beyond Line *to fade discoloration and further reduce age lines:*

1. Infiniti and Beyond Face Package, Anti-aging, Rosacea, Scars, Melasma *

2. Infiniti Primal Face Moisturizer

3. Infiniti Primal Face Package, Anti-aging, Rosacea, Scars, Melasma *

4. Infiniti Primal Face Serum

5. Infiniti Primal Face Toner

6. Personal Primal Package

Pomegranate Line is designed for dry skin and includes nourishing oils to hydrate the skin, maintain proper moisture, and prevent aging:

1. Pomegranate Primal Face Moisturizer

2. Pomegranate Primal Face Package, Norm-Dry *

3. Pomegranate Primal Face Serum

4. Pomegranate Primal Face Wash, Normal to Dry

HAIR

Products designed to clean and style hair while nourishing your hair and scalp:

1. Dirty Poo Primal Hair Package
2. Dirty Poo Primal Hair Wash
3. Primal Hair Serum, Coarse Hair Formula
4. Primal Hair Serum, Fine Hair Formula
5. Primal Hair Spray, Sweet
6. Primal Shampoo Bar, Lavender
7. Sea Salt Texturizing Spray, Salty
8. Shampoo Bar Primal Hair Package
9. Sweet & Salty, Primal Hair Styling Package

MAKEUP

100 percent natural and nourishing clays, foods, flowers, and herbs combined to create unique colors derived from hibiscus, beet root, spirulina, cocoa, alkanet root, cranberry, pink roses, and açaí berry:

1. Foundation (Cool, Warm)
2. Cheek Stain
3. Lid Stain
4. Primal Colors Packages
5. Professional Makeup Brushes

TEETH and GUMS

Products designed to help re-mineralize the teeth, prevent plaque formation, reduce inflammation, and improve gum tissue health.

1. Dirty Mouth Boost, Primal Gum Serum

2. Dirty Mouth Primal Package

3. Dirty Mouth Primal Toothpowder

PREGNANCY

Formulated to include only ingredients safe for pregnancy:

1. Primal Body Butter *

2. Primal Face and Body Package *

3. Sun-Up & Sun-Down Package *

4. Banished and Beyond Package for Acne *

5. Banished Primal Blemish Serum *

6. Banished Primal Face Mask for Acne *

7. Blossom Primal Belly Serum*

8. Grunt Primal Lip Balm *

9. Infiniti and Beyond Face Package, Anti-aging, Rosacea, Scars, Melasma *

10. Infiniti Primal Face Package, Anti-aging, Rosacea, Scars, Melasma *

11. Pomegranate Primal Face Package, Norm-Dry *

12. Primal Herbal-Clay Face Mask Anti-Aging

"I must rave about the Primal Toothpowder and Serum. I have never had a cavity in my life and in the past year, I had gone to the dentist to discover I had one in the early stages of development as well as some decay near the gum lines on a few of my teeth. The dentist wanted to drill my young cavity to prevent it from getting to a more severe stage and I declined. I was taking fermented cod liver oil twice a day and decided to floss twice a day and use the tooth powder and serum as my "toothpaste" for a few months and see what would result. I am proud to say that the decay on my gum lines is completely GONE and a follow-up visit to the dentist showed there was no longer development of a cavity—amazing! My teeth literally remineralized with the use of these incredible products. I'm never going back to conventional products again."

——Mara K.

Live Healthy.
Think Healthy.
Experience Health.

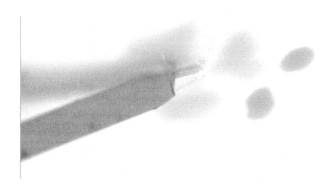

Banished Primal Blemish Serum

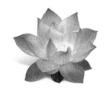

THE GREAT SKIN TRUTH

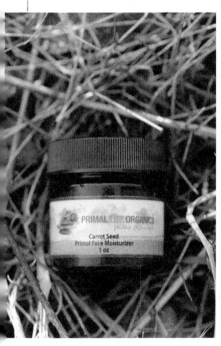

Carrot Seed Primal Face Moisturizer

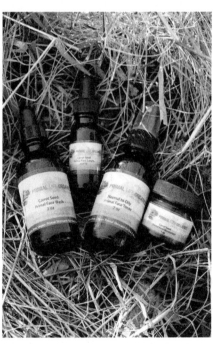

Carrot Seed Package

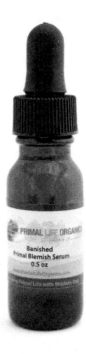

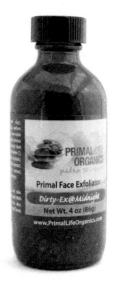

Primal Face Exfoliator

Banished Primal Blemish Serum

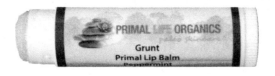

Grunt Primal Lip Balm

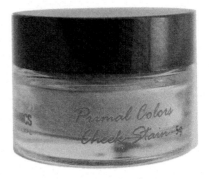

Primal Colors Cheek Stain

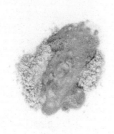

Primal Color Foundation
Medium Cool

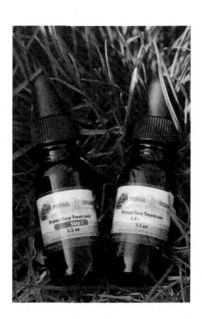

Primal Face Treatment
Fire and Ice

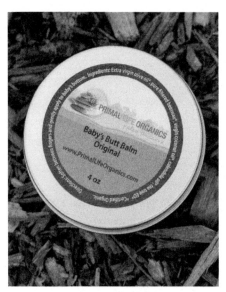

Primal Baby's Butt Balm

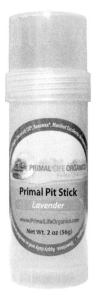

Stick Up
Lavender

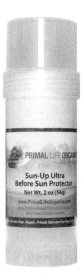

Sun-Up Ultra
Before Sun Protector

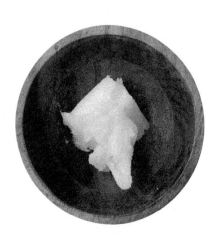

Sun-Down
After Sun Moisturizer

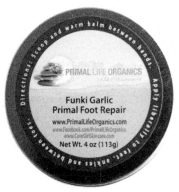

Funki Garlic
Primal Foot Repair

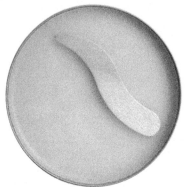

Funki Primal Foot Repair

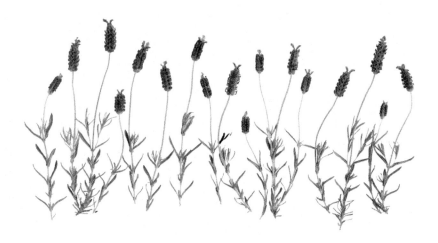

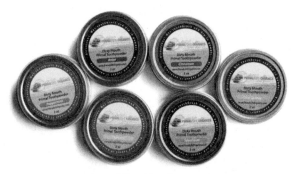

Dirty Mouth
Primal Toothpowder / 6 Flavors

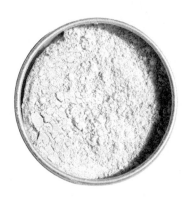

Dirty Mouth
Primal Toothpowder

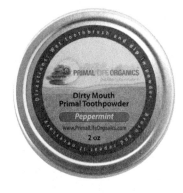

Dirty Mouth
Primal Toothpowder / Peppermint

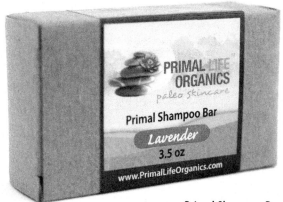

Primal Shampoo Bar
Lavender

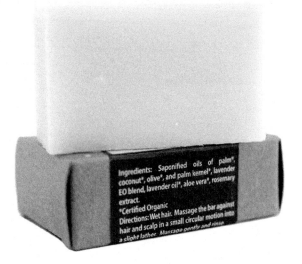

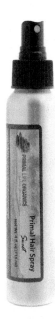

Primal Hair Spray
Sweet

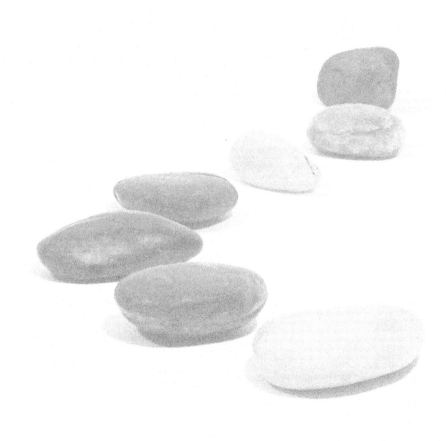

The Great Skin Talk

"Just wanted to say this is amazing. Nothing has ever worked for my skin. I have a lot of scarring and many hormonal breakouts. It's only been two weeks and I can see a HUGE difference. THANK YOU FOR CHANGING MY LIFE!"

—Jessica

"I absolutely love the Toothpowder and Gum Serum! My teeth feel super clean. I really like the PitStick too. First natural deodorant I've used that wasn't sticky and didn't have to be constantly reapplied to keep odor away."

—Lindsey R.

"I love love love the baby products. The cream has completely healed my son's reoccurring diaper rash and the spray is awesome!! Thanks for making an awesome product."

—Kelli D.

"I can't describe how much I love Fire & Ice. I use it once or twice a week and it's phenomenal. It makes my skin downright glow. I had been using other PLO products with great success before I got Fire & Ice, but once I got this, it made my skin better than I ever knew it could be. I didn't pull the trigger on this for a long time because of the price, but won't hesitate to reorder. It lasts a long time and the results are outstanding. Worth every penny and then some!"

—Julia

"The Torn Up is absolutely amazing at healing your skin. As a Cross-Fit athlete, I purchased this product to use on skin lacerations, and for that purpose, it works wonders! Additionally, during the winter, I have been using Torn Up Primal Skin Repair on my dry, cracked lips and it seems to heal them overnight! Amazing!"

—Lauren

"My skin loves this stuff. I have had fairly severe acne most of my life, and like many others, have tried every product under the sun, including several medications. The philosophy behind the PLO products makes a lot of sense to me, and my skin is responding better to this stuff than anything I've ever tried. (So far I've tried the Banished and Beyond package, and the PitStick, which is my new favorite for a deodorant without aluminum). When I first received those tiny bottles in the mail, I thought for sure I'd been ripped off. But no, they were right; the concentrated formulas that aren't bloated with cheap fillers go a surprisingly long way. My face looks noticeably improved, and I feel better about what I am applying to my skin. I also tried the oil cleansing method on my own, and I like the PLO stuff a lot better. I will definitely be ordering more."

—Amy

"I probably sound like a paid shill for PLO (I wish :P), but I really can't stop singing the praises of Trina and her team! Every time I see a new product released I have to jump on it immediately and the two facial scrubs (Dirty Ex Package) are no exception. Wow, they make my skin feel so silky smooth and amazing! After only two weeks of sporadic usage, the texture of my face has noticeably improved. I spent over 15 years fighting my skin and suffering from cystic acne on a daily basis. This left me with large pores on my cheeks, innumerable acne scars and an uneven tone throughout. Dirty Ex Sweet Revenge (paired with Fire & Ice) has made such a difference and in so little time. I even have stopped wearing face powder (except a light dusting of Primal Colors Foundation to eliminate shine). Each use uses so little, so the containers will last me for months!"

—Erin C.

"I've been using Dirty Poo for a little over a month now and my relationship with my hair has totally changed! I wash it twice a week and even in between washings, even with working out, it still looks clean and fresh. I don't even have to use dry shampoo in between washings like I always did with No Poo and with traditional shampoo! Best of all my limp locks seem to be history! My hair feels clean and fresh and still has some body and bounce to it! A day or two before washing, if it gets a little limp, I just pin it back in a French twist and it still looks great. I've already ordered an eight ounce container of Dirty Poo because this will be my hair care of choice for quite some time to come! I'm also a big fan of the Dirty Mouth Toothpowder, which leaves my teeth bright and white and somehow cleaner then regular toothpaste. Of course, not eating sugar & grains helps a lot in this regard as well! And my facial skin is clearer and more vibrant than it's ever been with the Carrot Seed range of products. Overall, I'm really impressed with your skin food and think it makes a wonderful counterpoint to a Paleo diet and lifestyle regime. Thanks so much and keep up the great work!"

—Dr. Christa

"I have been using Dirty Mouth Toothpowder and Boost Gum Serum for the past eight months. I must tell you my teeth (and gums) were a mess when I found Primal Life Organics. I have a dental nightmare in my mouth from years of eating candy and poor dental habits. I am very familiar with the 'ping' you get in a tooth when a cavity is forming. I must say: my teeth and gums are in amazing shape since I made the switch to your products! So, imagine my surprise two weeks ago when I felt a 'ping' in my top left molar! I had been 'ping free' for the past eight months!! How could this be???

"I have to tell you what I did because it is my testament to your healing products!! Shocked, I could not even wrap my head around the idea of a toothache! So I did what any other Primal would do!! I put a good size amount of Dirty Mouth Toothpowder on my aching tooth and let it bathe in the minerals of the toothpowder until the saliva carried it away! I repeated this again, then applied a generous amount of gum serum to the tooth and gum and went to bed.

"I forgot about this incident until just today—three weeks later!! I never felt that 'ping' again!! The toothpowder and gum serum halted whatever process was starting in my tooth and healed the tissue!! I am truly amazed and so thankful for your Dirty Mouth Package!! Thank you!!"

—Pingless-Vanessa in Washington!

"Funki Primal Foot Repair is the best stuff ever! This product has worked great for me after lots of barefoot beach walking, and just hanging most of the day on the beach or in the hotel. I really like to rub it on my feet before going to sleep or put socks on after applying (feels SO GOOD). This product also works well if you do barefoot gardening, river tubing trips, parks, rope swings, cliff jumping, snowboarding, skiing, running, hiking, or anything that tends to leave your feet a little beat up and tender. You will no longer need nasty athlete's foot spray; this cleared up my athlete's foot quickly. This also works great on cracking and dried out feet. Simply amazing product I will DEFINITELY continue to use and HIGHLY recommend this."

—Joe

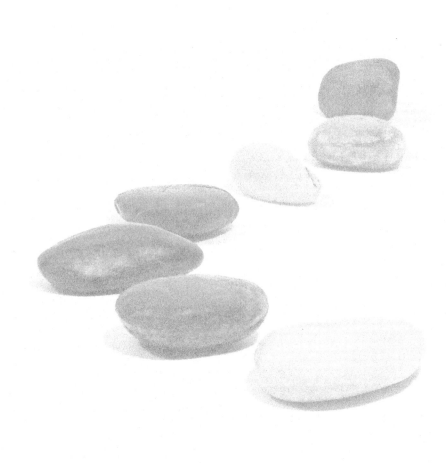

Recommended Online
Paleo Resources

Environmental Working Group (EWG)
Skin Deep http://www.ewg.org/skindeep

Purely Primal Skincare, written by Liz Wolfe NTP with Guest
Expert Trina Felber http://bit.ly/WCXWdJ
Purely Primal Skincare is a complete road map for information
on addressing skin issues and achieving results on the outside
by taking care of the body from the inside. *Purely Primal
Skincare* targets nutritional wellness, gut health, and dietary
supplementation as well as smart, non-toxic topical strategies to
improve acne, address skin conditions and improve the look of
hair, nails and teeth naturally!

Real Food Liz http://www.realfoodliz.com
Liz Wolfe is a Nutritional Therapy Practitioner (NTP™) certified
by the Nutritional Therapy Association and the best-selling author
of *Eat the Yolks* and *Purely Primal Skincare.* She is a nutrition coach,

podcaster, and magazine columnist, and she created the online cooking community Good Food for Bad Cooks. Liz focuses on nourishing and healing the body and skin from the inside-out using real food and holistic health principles.

This is so good... http://www.thisissogoodhome.com/
A Paleo/Primal/Ancestral Health centered blog where we explore healthful living through preparing and eating real food, exercising and maintaining physical fitness, reconnecting with nature, seeking out natural home and beauty options, and enjoying life! We create and share delicious grain/gluten-free recipes, discuss navigating through conventional medicine to find natural healthcare alternatives, and experiment with natural home and beauty products and DIY.

Tiffany Dalton Nutrition Solutions
http://www.glutenfreewithtiffany.com
Tiffany specializes in helping those with food sensitivities, digestive functioning, weight management, and autoimmune conditions. She offers Paleo friendly nutrition programs and nutritional consulting utilizing a functional medicine approach.

Cassy Joy's Fed+Fit http://www.fedandfit.com
A Paleo-friendly resource that specializes in empowering healthy lifestyle transformations through clear nutrition science, delicious and approachable recipes, one-on-one nutrition consulting, and corporate wellness program design.

Paleo Living Magazine http://www.PaleoMagazine.com
Paleo Living Magazine offers Paleo recipes, advice, informative

articles and interviews from top doctors and Paleo practitioners, and everything else you need to start or maintain your Paleo lifestyle. You can read our professionally designed monthly magazine on the iPad, iPhone or Android device or catch up on the huge amount of other articles and recipes on our blog.

Au Naturale Nutrition http://www.AuNaturaleNutrition.com
A holistic wellness website with educational articles about health, plus delicious, paleo, whole food recipes. Using the power of nutrition to become your most beautiful self, from the inside out!

Wholistic Boutique http://www.wholisticboutique.com
Wholistic Boutique is an on line holistic health coaching practice. We are a Health and Wellness Website. It is our passion to inspire, educate and ultimately transform people's lives through clean, green living. We also offer individually based healthy meal planning among other countless contributions to healthy body, healthy mind!

Fife Chiropractic & Health Awareness Center
http://www.fifechiropractic.com
A center for health that educates and treats for the three main causes of disease; thoughts, traumas, and toxins through nutrition and diet counseling, chiropractic, massage, decompression therapy, neuroemotional work, and lifestyle workshops.

Nourishing Excellence Nutritional Therapy LLC
*http://www.NourishingExcellence.com
As a Certified Nutritional Therapy Practitioner (NTP), my passion is to empower others to achieve optimal health and vitality

through targeted nutrition and lifestyle strategies.* Regardless if we're addressing hormonal issues, digestive health, fat loss, or other health concerns, I employ a diverse set of testing and evaluation modalities to develop a comprehensive wellness plan *unique to the individual*. As a first step, a complementary 15-minute initial consultation is welcome and encouraged! *

BH Sales http://www.kennelkelp.com/
BH Sales offers Creative Solutions for Holistic Health Care Products Distribution, featuring Kennel Kelp The World's Finest Nutrient Laden Supplement. BH Sales also offers Paleo Foods, skin care vitamins and supplements, Sacred Clay, organic soil amendments, green and raw food alternatives, and many other natural alternative health care products for both human and animal health.

Paleo Parents http://www.PaleoParents.com
Books:
> *Eat Like a Dinosaur*
> *Beyond Bacon*
> *Real Life Paleo*

Other Website Favorites

http://www.theprimalpalate.com

http://www.liveto110.com

http://www.marksdailyapple.com

http://thehealthyapple.com

http://www.ThePaleoMom.com

http://www.flametofork.com

http://paleobosslady.com

http://theprimalparent.com

http://www.paleoonthego.com

http://www.eatyourbeets.com

http://www.caterpillarfitness.com

http://paleomagazine.com

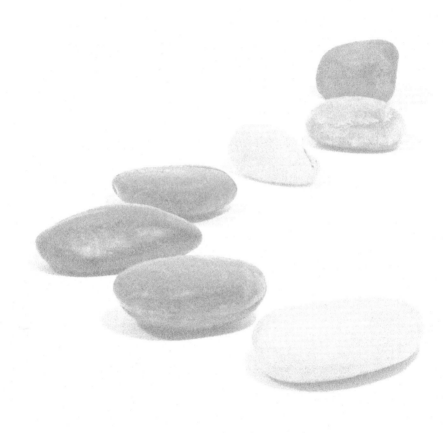

About the Author

When Trina Felber, RN, BSN, MSN, and Certified Registered Nurse Anesthetist (CRNA), discovered during her first pregnancy that all her high-end skincare products were loaded with toxic ingredients that could hurt her and her growing baby, she was shocked. Why didn't these products carry warning labels? Worse, why hadn't she read these labels before? Knowing that the skin is the largest organ in the body and the body's first line of defense, she began a quest in 2007 for organic and all-natural skincare products safe to use during pregnancy, only to learn there were none! Combining her outrage, medical knowledge, and Paleo philosophy with extensive research on natural, organic ingredients, she created Primal Life Organics skin-food, a complete line of quality skincare products that don't just moisturize, clean or rejuvenate, they actually feed your skin and all the cells of your body with the nutrients to create optimum health. Trina has appeared as a guest on America's Premier Experts® presentation of Health and Wellness Today, a television program seen on various ABC, CBS, NBC and Fox affiliates throughout the country. Trina is also the Guest Expert in Purely Primal Skincare written by Liz Wolfe, NPT.

Trina and her husband, Josh reside in Akron, Ohio with their daughter, Mia, and their twin sons, Cash and Roman.

Additional information about Trina Felber and her company can be found at: http://www.PrimalLifeOrganics.com.

CPSIA information can be obtained
at www.ICGtesting.com
Printed in the USA
BVOW11s2038300316

442376BV00018B/148/P